T0196199

A Patient's Voice

Inspiring And Practical Advice About Living With Chronic Health Conditions, Such As Cancer & Sarcoidosis, And Achieving Positive Results Regarding ALL Of Your Health Care Needs –
All Written From A Patient's Perspective and Personal Experiences!

Gilbert Barr, Jr.

iUniverse, Inc.
New York   Bloomington

A Patient's Voice
Inspiring And Practical Advice About Living With Chronic Health
Conditions, Such As Cancer & Sarcoidosis, And Achieving Positive
Results Regarding ALL Of Your Health Care Needs – All Written
From A Patient's Perspective and Personal Experiences!

iUniverse books may be ordered through booksellers or by contacting:

iUniverse
1663 Liberty Drive
Bloomington, IN 47403
www.iuniverse.com
1-800-Authors (1-800-288-4677)

ISBN: 978-1-4401-1988-0 (pbk)
ISBN: 978-1-4401-1989-7 (ebk)

Printed in the United States of America

iUniverse rev. date: 1/20/2009

THIS BOOK IS DEDICATED TO...

THE LOVING MEMORY OF MY BELOVED MOTHER-IN-
LAW
IDA BELLE McGHEE
...DECEMBER 26, 1940 – JULY 10, 2005...
YOU WERE THE BEST MOTHER-IN-LAW A SON-IN-LAW
COULD EVER WISH FOR!
UNTIL WE MEET ON THE OTHER SIDE...CIAO FOR NOW!

THE LOVING MEMORY OF MY BELOVED FATHER
GILBERT LEE BARR, SR.
...JUNE 19, 1926 – APRIL 26, 2006...
YOU WERE THE EPITOME OF WHAT A FATHER SHOULD
BE AND GUIDED ME EVERYDAY OF MY LIFE TO BE
THE SON, HUSBAND, FATHER, FRIEND, AND MOST
IMPORTANT, MAN FOR WHICH I'VE BECOME! WORDS
COULD NEVER ACCURATELY DESCRIBE MY LOVE FOR
YOU OR HOW MUCH I MISS YOU, SO I'LL JUST SAY...
"DADDY, I LOVE YOU!"

THE LOVING MEMORY OF MY BELOVED
GRANDMOTHER-IN-LAW
ROBERTA PAINE
...JULY 28, 1915 – JANUARY 5, 2007...
EVERYTIME I WATCH A COURT SHOW YOU WILL ENTER
MY MIND!
I'LL FOREVER TREASURE THE TIME WE SPENT
TOGETHER!

THE LOVING MEMORY OF MY LIFELONG FRIEND AND
WAS LIKE A BROTHER
LESTER "LEP" HOLMES
...MARCH 30, 1958 – SEPTEMBER 5, 2007...
NO MATTER WHAT YOU WERE A TRUE FRIEND AND
BROTHER! YOU WILL ALWAYS LIVE ON IN MY HEART!
REST IN PEACE MY BROTHER...I LOVE YOU!

THE LOVING MEMORY OF MY COUSIN-IN-LAW
SHERI KAYE SPRADLEY
...DECEMBER 4, 1963 – NOVEMBER 17, 2007...
YOU GAVE IT YOUR ALL AND WERE A TRUE FIGHTER
UNTIL THE END! YOUR FIGHTING SPIRIT IS AN
INSPIRATION TO US ALL!

THE LOVING MEMORY OF A DEAR FAMILY FRIEND
JENISE "GIGI" JONES
...JULY 26, 1963 – SEPTEMBER 12, 2008...
YOU WERE A WONDERFUL LIFELONG FRIEND TO MY
WIFE AND TO OUR FAMILY! YOU WILL BE GREATLY
MISSED – BUT NEVER FORGOTTEN!

There are four things that appear on every tombstone. (1) Your
Name; (2) Your Birthdate; (3) The Date Of Your Death; (4) And
The Only Thing That Really Counts..."The Dash"! Make Sure
Your Dash Will Be Remembered As A Positive And Fulfilling
Experience While You Still Have The Opportunity To Make A
Difference!!!

-

Contents

Intro
Why This Book?

Let me start by formally introducing myself. My name is Gilbert Lee Barr, Jr., born February 28, 1958, the only son to Gilbert and Georgia Barr in the rural North Florida town of Perry. I had a wonderful set of parents, who were both school teachers, my mother in elementary school and my father in high school, along with coaching football and basketball. I had a rather normal childhood, especially from a health perspective. I graduated high school in 1976 and went on to graduate from North Florida Junior College in June 1978.

I moved to Tallahassee, Florida in September 1978 and on to Detroit, Michigan in October 1985 where, as of 2009, I still reside. Growing up I was actively involved in sports, primarily basketball, and aside from odd jobs, worked as a computer operator until moving to Detroit. There I was employed with Electronic Data Systems (EDS), where I spent the majority of my time with the corporation supporting a national health care claims system in a variety of areas until leaving the corporate world in April 2002, primarily due to health reasons. I have been with my wife, Ma-Shelle, since 1990 and have one stepdaughter, Ra-Shelle, and one granddaughter, Saniya. I am the sole author of this book, which is based on my life, beliefs, experiences and opinions. To ensure we are on the same page and you benefit from reading this book I want to give you upfront my primary objectives and disclaimers.

This book is written from three viewpoints. The first is strictly from a patient's perspective. The writings are solely based on my personal experiences as a patient, caregiver, and interactions with the medical community, along with those others in my life. Any information is based on my opinions obtained from my experiences and things I've learned over the years. Unless noted, no information in this book is from a medical professional's perspective and by no means whatsoever is intended as medical advice. Always consult your medical professionals before applying any information acquired outside of your medical professionals to your daily life.

The second viewpoint is from my professional experience supporting a national health care claims system for over 16 years. The system supported the benefits for corporations such as GM, Ford, Chrysler, and K-Mart, to name a few. I worked in a variety of positions such as data center manager for multiple data centers, data center project manager, developed financial forms, financial analyst responsible for the data, printing and mailing of financial forms to customers, and as a business analyst responsible for implementing policy updates, supporting current policies and troubleshooting any issues regarding the processing of claims. This experience allows me to understand what goes on behind the scenes with claims processing from a professional perspective. In addition I have been in the position where I depend on health care benefits for my own health situation for over 20 years. As a result I can relate both the professional and personal perspectives of health care benefits.

The third viewpoint, and most influential, for which this book is written is based on my personal faith in God. Faith is an important part of my life and has a major impact on everything I do, thus my faith cannot be ignored as having an impact on the writing of this book and my actions during my life in general. I want to make it perfectly clear I have no intention to convert or influence anyone in his/her personal beliefs. I have no alternative motives other than giving you insight on what I believe and how my beliefs have helped me get through life, especially my health life, in a positive manner, as they simply can not be ignored.

I'm not going to dwell on my personal philosophy regarding my beliefs because I feel strongly that is a personal choice for each individual. However, I will tell you the basis of my spiritual philosophy is quite simple and pure. I believe in the unconditional worship of one God for everyone. It is my belief all people are created equal in the image of God. If we weren't equal, why are humans able to reproduce and why is everyone susceptible to the same diseases regardless of his/her personal traits or beliefs?

It doesn't matter to me, nor should it to you, how an individual gets to God, as that is once again a personal choice. At the end of the day the same God is the Master of us all. It is your personal responsibility and duty to face God on your judgment day and only God can judge your actions on earth. I feel if you treat everyone with equal respect, pray every day, and when you do wrong – as all humans do from time to time – you take responsibility for your actions, sincerely repent of your sins to God, and seek forgiveness of those your actions have offended, then, you will be okay on your judgment day.

For the sake of this book, and a primary source of my actions, the emphasis will be on your inner voice which we all have. Whether you call it your inner voice, gut feeling, instinct or fate, I strongly believe your inner voice is God communicating with you and guiding you. How many times have you listened to your inner voice and good has followed your actions or you have not listened to your inner voice and a bad decision resulted? We are placed in situations for a reason. It's up to the individual to have the trust in his/her faith to follow that inner voice. It's my faith in God that has allowed me over the years to trust unconditionally in my inner voice to guide me throughout every aspect of my life. This is why faith cannot be omitted as a source for my viewpoints and experiences.

My overall objectives are to help other medical patients (hereon referred to as patients), caregivers, medical professionals, family members, employers, and the general public to learn from my vast experiences dealing with chronic health conditions. I understand from experience that living with any medical condition affects all aspects of one's life. I want to give my experiences on how to be a successful patient or caregiver to others so they too will be successful and have the benefit of someone's prior experience, knowledge, and tips which I lacked in the beginning of my health journey. I understand everyone is a unique individual and in turn handles his/her own situations in a unique way, but hopefully I can help you develop your own beneficial processes from the simple tips I provide. There are a lot of things that's going to be written that might sound simplified or like plain ole common sense but when you're sick or helping a loved one and the stress levels rise, these simple tips or actions can be easily forgotten. My objective is to instill those processes into your memory bank so when the situation arises you will be prepared.

I don't expect that everything I discuss, all of my advice, or the influence of my beliefs to be relative or perceived by everyone. Instead, it is my objective for each and every one of my readers to relate to some aspect of this book, to learn from other aspects about which they might not have thought and after completion to have developed a better understanding of how you, too, can live a positive life, regardless of your personal or health situation.

As I discuss my life going from a healthy young man to where I am today healthwise, there are going to be negative aspects which I must address. To avoid any misunderstanding that may give the wrong impression or cause the message about living a positive life in the face of adverse circumstances, here are a few disclaimers to ensure we are still on the same page.

I believe in speaking my mind in a direct and blunt fashion. Life is like a roller coaster for which positive/negative, good/bad, joy/pain, richer/poorer, happiness/depression, wellness/sickness, and life/death are thrown at us throughout our lifetime. How we address, and react to those situations determines our quality of life. Life provides us with no dress rehearsals! The trick is dealing with the negative for what it is.

Please understand, without a shadow of a doubt, I have absolutely no complaints about how my life has been nor do I feel any bitterness toward any situation I've encountered. I'll admit in the past I had a lot of bitterness but as I evolve as a man I've been able to put those feelings to rest. All of my experiences make me who I am today and who I will be in the future. It is what it is and it was what it was so the only choice I have is to look my reality square in the face. Do not interpret the fact I'm writing about negative aspects of my life to be me feeling sorry for myself, looking for pity, blaming others or whining. The whole purpose of writing about and addressing negative situations, like the positive experiences, is to give you the whole picture and an understanding of how to deal with negative situations in order to turn them positive. Without the negatives in life there can be no positives. My objective is to have you benefit from my experiences and avoid some of the same negatives I've experienced in life. My message and my attitude, regardless of the situation or perception, are always positive. Please never lose sight of that fact!

I've learned from my past writings and conversations there are usually three ways people can react to negative situations. The first is to ignore it because you don't believe such a thing could happen to you or your family. I beg of you do not take this approach in life because negatives need to be addressed in order to obtain positive results. How many times have you heard a newscast where a terrible situation has taken place and a witness says, "I can't believe this happened here because nothing like this ever happens around here?" Just because something hasn't happened or never happened to you doesn't mean it doesn't happen to others or may in the future affect your life.

If your 3-year-old child gets into a fight every time he/she is around other kids at day care, on playgrounds or at any social gathering where kids play together, you must acknowledge and address that there's a problem with your child's behavior. You won't ignore the fact your child is getting into fights every single time he/she plays with other children just because you personally have never been in a fight your entire life. No, you'll address why the fights are occurring, and how to correct the situation to turn your child's playtime into a positive experience, for him/her and the other children. Facing negative situations helps you deal with the situations if or when they affect your life. You are only as prepared as your own ability to face reality with an open mind!

When I first met my wife and we would have to make a decision, she would tell me I was negative because of the process I used to make a decision that would affect my family or me. I always ask myself three questions and if the answer to all three isn't "yes" then I probably won't go with the decision. First I think of the worst thing that could possibly happen if I go with the decision and ask myself, "Can I handle the consequence?" Next I think of the most rewarding and positive outcome of going with this decision (sometimes you can get more than you bargain for) and again ask myself, "Can I handle the consequence?" Last, I think of any and every possibility in between and then ask the same question once again, "Can I handle the consequences?" If my answers are "yes", I go with the decision. If not, I rethink the decision until I can achieve "yes" as the answer three times over.

When I first started discussing our decisions and this process out loud she immediately accused me of being a negative person simply because I prepared myself for the worst. I didn't hope for the worst, or have the attitude the worst was going to happen, or even think it would occur. I just wanted to understand if it did I could handle it. However as time went on she started to understand I wasn't being negative but instead was preparing myself to turn any possible result positive and make good decisions in life. Discussing or preparing for negative events doesn't make you a negative or whining person but instead is one step in many to living a positive quality of life. Don't put on blinders and ignore negative situations because you don't want to deal with them. In the end they aren't going away and could cause you avoidable heartache/hardships.

The second way I've seen people react to negative situations brought out by myself always puts a big smile on my face. This method of handling negative situations is to blame me personally for discussing them, calling me a whiner or complainer. In turn they force their negative energy on me and start realizing how positive their situation or their loved ones are. "Gil is so negative. I deal with my situation so much better. I have newfound respect for my caregiver and all they do for me because they never complain." they might comment. In other words they have used me as a punching bag to discover the positives in their life, which is fine with me because that's my objective.

It's like selling your home. You need to sell the home for $200,000 in order to pay your bills and move somewhere else. Therefore you put the home on the market for $250,000 expecting to negotiate down. The buyer comes back with a forceful offer stating they will only pay $220,000, final offer. You think about it, or as business folks do pretend like you're thinking about it, then come back and accept the offer. The buyers' walks away feeling positive about themselves because they drove a hard bargain and got you to come down $30,000, where in reality you actually got what you wanted plus $20,000.

If you can look at others and discover the positive in your own life, then that's just another way of using negative situations to create positive results for your life. Of course you're going in the backdoor to achieve this objective but at least you've achieved it.

The last way, and the way I hope you will react to any negative situations in this book, or your own life, is to look at the situation as it is, then, in turn, discover how to either avoid the situation or if you have experienced it, understand how to turn it positive. I promise you everything I've experienced is true and not hyped in anyway for the sake of this book. I have no intention of blaming anyone associated with any negative situation or experience I've encountered nor am I personally attacking any person or profession with my comments, solutions, or opinions. Everything is intended to turn negative situations into positive experiences by addressing and dealing with them head on. It's my hope you will read this book with an open mind and thus obtain a positive attitude. This is my primary objective, regardless of the situation or experience.

I want to be bluntly honest with you here. If addressing negative situations are too much for you to handle or you're the type of person who has a closed mind and feels your life, beliefs and way of life is the only way, immediately close this book and return it to the place you bought it for a refund. This book is not for you! On the other hand, if you're able to listen to other experiences, beliefs and opinions with an open mind and you're looking to get insight from another patient's perspective regarding how to live a positive life within your own or a loved one's health situation, you should find this book of value. Keep reading!

Now before we get started, I want to reiterate this book is based, unless otherwise noted, on my personal experiences as a patient/caregiver, beliefs and opinions. Understanding the source of any information you obtain is the most important thing you must do in order to determine if the information is worth using. For example, if you want advice on how to build a successful marriage who would you rather consult, someone who has been successfully married for 25 years or a single person? If you want advice on how to successfully raise a child do you listen to a parent of four or someone planning to have their first baby? If you're in the air taking your first test flight as a pilot who do you want sitting next to you, someone with over 20 years of actual flight experience or someone with four years of college and only has experience on a flight simulator? If you're going to follow the findings of a study regarding a type of food, first find out who funded the study and what they had to gain or lose from the results. Get my point? Bottom line…all of the information in this book is based on my actual experiences and beliefs. Never lose track of that fact.

I sincerely hope my experiences and the knowledge I've obtained from those experiences over the course of my life will be of value to your life. If you're still reading this book then hopefully we are on the same page in regard to my objectives. So without further ado, open your mind and let's get started.

1
The Ups And Downs Of Life

I didn't start out life as someone who could be entitled a "Professional Patient". No, it was a long and painful experience, literally and figuratively, physically and mentally, financially and emotionally! For those of you who have read my two previous books, the first two chapters will sound familiar as I tell my story, although a lot has changed since my last book was released in 2004. I hope you will still come away with something new that will make your life more positive. For those who haven't – here is my story.

From 1958 through 1985 I lived a normal life from a health perspective. I had a couple broken bones, colds, too many jammed fingers to count, and a wet sinus problem due to my allergic reaction to the pollen generated by the pine trees that were everywhere in Taylor County. I played basketball practically everyday, sometimes more than once, and swam regularly as well. I was at the top of my game physically and in the prime of my life. However once I moved to Detroit things changed immediately.

The first noticeable change was with my sinus problems, as they changed from wet mucus to hard mucus making it at times difficult to breathe. As a result I started developing migraine headaches, which I must admit were extremely painful.

My migraines were very unique and specific in the fact they would only occur in the left corner of my right eye. At first I could tolerate them but as time went on they got to the point I had to stop everything I was doing because I just couldn't function, as they would last anywhere from a couple of hours to over 12 hours. When they were active it felt as if someone was applying pressure directly to a nerve, similar to when a dentist touches an exposed nerve before the Novocain has had time to start working, only the dentist continued to apply pressure. Then without warning they would immediately stop, and when I say immediately, I mean immediately! It was the greatest sensation I have ever felt but yet amazing at the same time.

Throughout 1986 the migraines continued and I did my best to tolerate them. By 1987 they were occurring at least once a week. As it was about to turn out my migraines were only a small piece of the puzzle God was getting ready to place me in. I was about to encounter a major test of Faith. In January 1987 a dramatic event took place in my life and without warning my future changed.

When I moved to Detroit my girlfriend of five years, Cynthia Vanessa Reese, came with me. On a cold night in January we went to bed around 11:00 o'clock. We had a long talk about how lucky we were to have each other and how good we got along, as we were not only lovers but best friends as well, with plans to marry in June. She went to the restroom, came back to bed and we both said to each other, "I love you." The next morning I woke up, Vanessa didn't! She died in her sleep at the age of 27as a result of Pulmonary Emboli, which the doctor described as a shower of blood clots (more than five) to the lungs at one time. Needless to say my world was turned upside down in a stop of a heartbeat.

I spent 1987 grieving and at the same time dealing with the migraines, which were now causing me to vomit mucus on a regular basis as well. I played them off as part of the grieving process but deep down I knew something wasn't right. Since I had never been sick before I didn't understand how to get the help I needed as the doctors seemed unconcerned.

Around the end of 1987, although I still missed Vanessa greatly, I knew life went on and I too had to start focusing on living. Aside from the migraines and vomiting on what was now almost a daily basis, other symptoms started to occur as well. I started to experience extreme thirst and a strong sensation to urinate frequently. Neither of these symptoms were anything like I had ever experienced and both were so strong it would feel as if you would go into shock if the need was not satisfied. To this day I still can't accurately articulate the feelings.

As a result of the symptoms I was experiencing my appetite started to decrease causing me to have a constant drop in weight. My energy levels were making it difficult to do basic everyday functions such as going to work or hanging out with friends. It was getting where even playing basketball, a major part of my life, was too much as I would usually vomit after a few games and have to stop playing. Around this time blood started to accompany the mucus which I was throwing up. At times not only was it a painful experience but could be a messy one as well. I started keeping extra shirts in my cubical at work in case I messed one up during the day and I always wore white shirts, hoping no one would notice if I changed shirts during the day. My health was now changing my everyday quality of life in more ways than one.

From 1988 through 1989 other symptoms started to appear such as skin problems. The skin problems were two-fold with one affecting my face, as it started to become two-toned in no specific pattern. The other symptom was skin poison which consisted of itching red blisters covering my arm. This struck me as weird since growing up in Florida I had never even used sunscreen without problems, and now I was getting sun poison just driving my car. The mental aspect of these health changes was starting to take a major toll on me.

Anyone who has experienced health problems, especially mysterious symptoms with no positive results or diagnosis, will tell you the mental aspect of your situation outweighs the physical pain. The fear of the unknown and subliminal denial that your health is deteriorating can cause depression. You are in trouble once you start giving in to the mental pressure. For me, this is when I put my faith in God and continue to live life to the best of my ability and circumstances, although I must admit it was getting harder each and every day as the symptoms continued to mount.

Other symptoms included a constant cough that would sometime produce mucus coming out of my mouth with no warning, an embarrassing situation when this happened in public. Eventually I couldn't even finish a sentence without coughing and talking on the phone, a major part of my job, became almost impossible. My feet also became rough and cracked, especially my heels, while parts of my body were turning a yellow tone. Muscle cramps in my feet, calves, sides, and hands were everyday events as well. Most mornings I would wake up to blood on my pillow as nose bleeds were becoming a common occurrence in my ever changing health life.

In fact from 1988 until 1991 I never slept more than two hours at a time due to having to urinate and get something to drink, usually followed by vomiting. During the day I would constantly vomit on a regular basis and fight pain, thirst, and the frequent and sometimes painful need to urinate. This was now an everyday routine.

I now understood how individuals can hide illnesses because I became a pro at it. I could be sitting in a meeting, excuse myself, go to the restroom, vomit, put some peppermint in my mouth, and return to the meeting as if nothing happened. Unless it was one of those times where I had to struggle to breath and thus was noisy, no one ever had a clue. I did this for years!

In reality it wasn't that transparent as my looks changed dramatically, my ability to play basketball or work a normal schedule was obvious to everyone but me, and my personality was changing as well. I did everything I could to avoid people whenever possible. It's a wonder my employer never drug tested me because I started looking like a well-kept crack head with a lot of the characteristics. At this point life was going in a downward swing and dealing with the simple things in life became overwhelming for me. But wait - there's more!

Dental issues too became a problem as my crowns were coming off on a regular basis and cavities were popping up more than usual. There were a couple of incidents with my dentist that were unusual, to say the least. As I was having my crown re-set I would have to wait about five minutes for the cement to harden. Usually during this time saliva is normally pouring down my chin but when the dentist removed the cotton and told me to spit, absolutely no saliva was present in my mouth! We just kind of looked at each other like we were in the twilight zone until he gave me some mouthwash and told me to rinse.

Thinking back this should have been a clear sign something wasn't normal but instead I just went on with my life, still mentally battling what was physically going on while at the same time thinking everything would clear up eventually. Being sick or having a chronic health condition wasn't something with which I was familiar nor obviously knew how to handle, except to acknowledge, yet at the same time deny. Depression continued to ease into my life as I struggled mentally with the unknown.

Finally, around the beginning of 1989 something positive happened when I laid eyes on a beautiful woman who literally made my heart melt at first sight. She was a waitress at a local restaurant I frequented for lunch, and I knew immediately I wanted a relationship with her. The problem was how to make a relationship with her a reality.

You see when you're sick, especially experiencing an unexplainable downward swing, starting or maintaining relationships, either personal or business, is a very difficult task and something, quite frankly, I wanted to avoid. It's hard enough dealing with relationships in a successful manner when you're healthy! Approaching someone I wanted to start a relationship with was a chance I wasn't prepared to take. What if she said no? What did I have to offer her anyway? It would be unfair for me to expect a woman to start a relationship with someone who is sick and based on how I felt I didn't have the energy to put into a relationship anyway. I told myself, "Oh well, I can always dream. If it's meant to be then it's meant to be. God will lead her to me." And that's exactly what, as God always does when the chips are down, happened!

Fortunately we ended up exchanging phone numbers. Her name was Ma-Shelle (pronounce Michelle) and we hit it off from the start. My life finally had something positive to live for! If not for my strong faith in God, and now with Ma-Shelle in my life, well, I don't know what kind of life I would have now, if any life at all. Yes, it had gotten that bad, especially from a mental perspective, and I didn't see how it could get any worse. Of course I was wrong once again!

Other symptoms started to become present such as male hormone issues that included having problems with erections, not producing semen, my testicles started to shrink, my facial hair was thinning out, and my breast started to enlarge slightly. For a man in his early 30's who had finally found a woman he loved and wanted to spend his life with, these issues were a major concern in my life with seemingly nowhere to turn. This isn't something you talk about with the fellows in the locker room or around the office cooler. Fortunately my relationship with Ma-Shelle was open enough that she was able to keep my sanity positive. Reflecting back it might have been a positive turn of events as we built our relationship on open communications and friendship as opposed to just a sexual priority relationship.

To add to the problems I became very sensitive to the touch to the point even a sheet on my feet or Ma-Shelle putting her arm around me was painful. By 1990 I was a mess both physically and even more so mentally!

You might have asked yourself by now what were the doctors saying about all of these symptoms? Well, this is one of those situations where you turn negative experiences into knowledge so you can learn how to obtain positive results in the future because there was nothing positive about my experiences with the seven doctors I encountered between 1986 and 1990. For those of you who don't want to hear about negative situations or are naïve to reality, wake up to the real world because it was what it was!

Before I continue let me say, right or wrong, looking in hindsight with a more educated outlook on being a patient and the medical environment, I take partial responsibility for the results. I was in a strange world and didn't know how or when to advocate for myself. Plus when you're sick, but in denial at the same time, when you hear what you want to hear you're satisfied, even though your inner voice is telling you its wrong and your symptoms continue to worsen. That's just human nature, although it's a bad human trait we all must consciously fight, especially when you're sick.

I didn't even know how to pick a doctor, as in the past I had never been in this situation. Living in Perry - a small rural town - or in Tallahassee, which was just an hour away from Perry, I automatically used the doctor my parents used. To help me in this situation, since I was over a thousand miles from my Perry doctor, I would get referrals from other people with whom I worked with. The problem was they were usually young, healthy, or just moved to Detroit as I had. You must always ensure your referrals have used the doctor as you need them, again something I was unaware of at this time in my life.

With my coverage within a Health Maintenance Organization (HMO), the coverage my employer provided in the 1980s, I had to choose a doctor in a specific clinic. I would have a primary doctor who, if needed, would refer me to a specialist within the clinic. Bottom line is picking a doctor for me was like finding a needle in a haystack, only with consequences that would affect me for life.

Each doctor put me through the same routines with the same results - all seven of them! The routine consisted of a complete physical, chest X-ray, blood work, and a test for diabetes. Each and every time the result for all of the symptoms I've described was that I had a bad sinus problem, was given pain pills, and told that when the weather changed I would get better. Even though I saw several of the doctors through several weather changes with my symptoms worsening this was the diagnosis. Some told me most of my problems were mental and didn't really exist, especially the male hormone issues and migraine headaches. Not one of the seven doctors sent me to a specialist or ask for additional tests. Like I said, at this time in my inexperienced life I didn't know to ask, no demand, further tests or to be sent to a specialist. That's all a patient asked is honesty. If you don't know or your diagnosis isn't working ask for help. This was a learning experience for me that would not only benefit me in the future to "not" make the same mistakes but unfortunately this learning experience cost me dearly, for life.

Finally in 1990 the seventh doctor, after giving me the same diagnosis, had the solution - move back to Florida because the reason I had sinus problems was because there was no salt water in the air. Even after I explained to him there was no saltwater in the air where I grew up, plus for the last few years I had been using a saltwater solution for my sinuses and therefore I had been exposed to more saltwater than I ever had in Florida, he simply looked at me and asked me to whom he should write a letter so that I could be transferred to Florida doing the same job. I had moved to Detroit because my employer had no accounts in Florida for which I was qualified. For me that was the last straw on a pile that had been building for years!

I went home with my mind, hopes, and spirit totally out of commission. I remember getting down on my knees and praying to God to show me the way because I think I had reached my limit and I needed His help. As always God was listening and help came the very next day. Another example of how God puts everything in place even though at the time it might not be obvious to you.

I went to get my mail and there was a coupon for a free consultation at a local chiropractor's office. The coupon read, "Can help with back problems, auto accidents, headaches, …". Hmm, a light bulb went off in my head as headaches caught my mind's eye. My mother had been telling me she knew of people who went to a chiropractor for headaches with great results. However for me there were a couple of problems.

First, I have a deep fear of being adjusted and secondly my insurance didn't cover chiropractor visits. However for some reason, actually it was God subliminally guiding me, I didn't throw the coupon away with my other junk mail but instead put it on my dining room table. The very next day after my nightly migraine, vomiting, and other now normal routines I made an appointment to see the chiropractor for a free consultation.

In a few days I went to the free consultation and explained my over-all health situation, emphasizing the migraines, to the chiropractor. He was a young doctor, easy to talk to and seemed to pay close attention to what I was saying instead of acting like he already knew what I was going to say, which is what I had been accustomed to over the past five years. When I finished he asked if he could take a few X-rays, on the house of course, to see if he could see something that stood out. After a few minutes he came back and said, "It was just as I suspected. Let me ask you something. When you get the migraines does it feel as if there is pressure on a nerve in the corner of your eye, say like when you go to a dentist and they touch an exposed nerve?" This blew my mind because that was exactly as I described it in the past only this time I had only referred to it as a migraine, and not by the dentist example, during our conversation. "Yes," I replied, "that's exactly how it feels and then goes away instantly."

He went on to explain the top bone in my vertebrate was slightly off center. Therefore when the sinus cavity would fill up with hard mucus it would put pressure directly on the nerve affecting the left corner of my right eye. When the sinus cavity would finally drain the pressure would release thus the instant relief. To top it off my mother had a rough time giving birth to me, which is why I'm an only child. As a result of the rough birth the bone was probably off center my entire life. It wasn't until I moved to Detroit my mucus became hard in my sinus cavities and in turn my migraines started. With about six weeks of twice a week adjustments the bone should be straightened back to normal and the migraines should be history.

I couldn't believe my ears! After seven doctors and five years I was finally hearing an explanation from a medical professional explaining my migraines and a realistic solution. And to think this good news was coming from a chiropractor, who, at the time, those other so-called "knowledgeable doctors" didn't even consider on their level had figured out in one visit what they couldn't in several visits, and in some cases, years. There was still one slight problem. My insurance didn't cover chiropractor treatments.

Each treatment was going to cost $88 but since I didn't have insurance he would charge me $44 a treatment, nice of him but still a concern for my pocketbook. At $44 a treatment, twice a week for six weeks, it was going to cost me $528 out of pocket, still kind of steep for me at this time in my financial life. So I did what I recommend everyone do. I talked finances upfront and honestly. Never forget that just because it's a medical service doesn't mean a deal can't be worked out, no different than any other business. He told me to go talk to his office manager and after a brief discussion we came up with a deal of $22 a treatment, cash, for a total of $264 for all of the treatments.

I was still scared out of my mind the first treatment, as my fear of being adjusted was in the front of my mind. As I lay on my back he slowly rested my head in his hands just off the table. He slowly moved my head and neck, back and forth, relaxing me to the point I was in his control, almost in a trance. Without warning he popped my neck so fast all I could hear was "CRACK" and I immediately replied, "Damn!" and gave him a look as to say you have one second to get out of here before I jump off this table and …!!! He looked at me, smiled and said, "Gil, that will be your treatment but I'll never be able to get you perfectly again." When I realized my neck wasn't broken and still intact I looked up at him and laughed as I replied, "You can say that again." And he never did!

The rest of my treatments consisted of the neck popping from a variety of positions. He would put his fist hard into my spine up and down along with massaging my sinus cavities in my face. Since I didn't use any drugs I had no side effects except for soreness from the adjustment as if I had just played a few games of basketball. After six weeks my migraines were gone and to this day I've never experienced a migraine again! Excuse me while I go knock on wood.

Although the migraines were the most painful symptom I have ever experienced, I still had many other health problems. Not only were all of the previous symptoms still present and getting worse but it was getting where I would fall asleep at the drop of a hat, although I never fell asleep on the chiropractor's table. So I did something else, which I suggest everyone do regardless of the situation. When you find success with a resource and need additional help, ask the resource for a referral to someone they know and trust. Whether it's home improvement, a mechanic, sports, business, or whatever the situation, but even more so in the medical profession, remember this basic fact - successful people surround themselves with successful people. Positive resources keep people successful. No one person ever won a World Series, Super Bowl, or NBA Championship without a team. So I asked if he could recommend me to a doctor who could possibly help me. He suggested his own personal physician.

He called ahead to put in a good word for me and help get me an immediate appointment. The new doctor was easy to talk to as well and I gave him an earful. I think he took my case as a challenge. After all I did have some deep issues going on. After a few months of the same tests, with some different tests thrown in as well, he was still at a dead end and I was getting sicker as each week past. He did however give me what was called a "Six-Pack" which was basically cortisone pills where you took six pills the first day then reduced the dosage by one pill for six days. I could tell a slight difference in my ability to eat and sexual issues, however not enough to consider the medication a cure. Plus this type of medication was not intended as a long-term solution but as a way of keeping me going while my new doctor tried to figure out what was wrong with me. Frustration was starting to build on all parties involved and from a personal perspective my health was deteriorating at an even more rapid rate.

In February 1991 I had an appointment scheduled to review some tests I had taken the previous week. This was an appointment I'll never forget. As I entered the head nurse immediately called me back, before I could even sit down, and you know that doesn't happen at a doctor's office unless something serious is going on. I was taken to the doctor's personal office, as opposed to an examining room, another sign something out of the norm was getting ready to take place. The doctor came in a few minutes later and sat down with a serious look on his face. He began by saying, "Gil, I feel we have developed a good relationship between us so if you don't mind I'm going to be blunt". I shook my head to say yes. He continued, "At first I thought some of your symptoms might have been mental or from the traumatic loss of your girlfriend several years ago, but after getting to know you I don't think you have any mental issues at all, in fact just the opposite. After looking at all of your test results I can conclude that, although you do have some sinus problems, sinus problems are not causing your overall health problems. There is something however wrong with your pituitary gland, a small gland in your brain that controls your endocrine system, among a lot of other functions in your body. The problem is I don't know what's wrong or what to do about it. One thing I can say with confidence is if nothing is done I have no doubt in a few weeks you will fall asleep and not wake up. If nothing is done you are on a rapid direct course with death."

He paused, I guess to see how I was going to react. It's funny because what he was saying had little impact on me because I already knew by how I was feeling if nothing was done I was in trouble. Hell, I was already in trouble! Not to be macho but I'm not scared of death, as God will determine when it's time for me to come home, so having the term referred to in reference to me had no emotional or panic effect on me. Actually what went through my mind was it's probably time to tell my parents I'm seriously sick and I asked myself if it was fair to Ma-Shelle, and especially Ra-Shelle (Ma-Shelle's 6 year old daughter who was about to become my daughter as well), to start a new life with them if I wasn't going to be around much longer. I came out of those thoughts quickly, nodded and looked at him with a look that said, "I'm okay but what are you going to do to keep me alive?"

He continued to say, "I'm going to send you to an endocrinologist, one of the best in the business, and see if he can figure out what's causing all of your problems. I'll call ahead so you don't have to wait as a new patient because he has a very long waiting list. Please do not hesitate to call me anytime if you have any questions and let me know how it works out." I thanked him for being the first medical professional to be honest with me and admit he didn't know, and even more so for asking for help. I told him I would let him know what happened as we parted ways. When I got to my car I thanked God for finally giving me hope then went to see Ma-Shelle. I still didn't fully tell Ma-Shelle or my parents the seriousness of my conversation with the doctor. I figured they couldn't do anything about it anyway so why worry them. My inner voice kept telling me things would work out and with everything I had been through the past five years I had no where to go but up.

...1...

Just because I had bad experiences, and addressed them, with a few doctors doesn't mean all doctors are bad. No, there are a lot of doctors who are professional and exceptional. Look at it like the bad cop who beats a handcuffed suspect or a teacher who had inappropriate actions with a student. It doesn't mean the majority of police officers are abusive or the majority of teachers aren't trustworthy with your children. Here's the point - we, and even more importantly their peers, must acknowledge then address the problem directly so other situations will not occur. Please don't put on blinders to problems because if you do they will never be corrected!

2
A New Reality

The next week or so was hell mentally as I waited for my appointment with the endocrinologist. When the appointment came, although my frame of mind was hopeful and positive, it turned out to be once again frustrating. He had my chart but wanted to do a few more tests. I snapped at him by asking, "Don't you have my charts with the same tests already done?" He just smiled with an understanding smile and calmly told me he wanted to start his own chart. I scheduled a follow-up appointment for the next week and went to have what seemed like more of the same tests done. I have to admit I was full of attitude and frustrated mentally. I kept saying to myself, "Here I go again!" I was almost ready to fall asleep permanently but I knew God had other plans for me.

The next week I returned for the results, expecting more of the same. However this time I would finally get to the bottom of my problems. He came in and said it was just as he suspected. I flashed back to my chiropractor visit as this was what he said when he returned with my results as well. The endocrinologist told me I had sarcoidosis (pronounced sar-coy-do-sis). Sarcoidosis is an autoimmune disease that can affect any organ or gland in the body including the eyes, skin and spine in the form of granulomas, which are basically lumps that develop in organs or glands when cells from the immune system clump together for some unknown reason. Sarcoidosis can affect anyone regardless of race, sex, age, living or working environments, financial status, political affiliations, sense of humor or any other factor of which you can think. There's currently (2008) no known origin for the disease although several theories exist such as something in the environment causes the immune system to overreact, such as some type of bacteria, it could be genetic or maybe a combination of some type. We simply don't know for sure but strides are being made. There are no "standard" tests performed to detect sarcoidosis, as most times a biopsy is performed, nor is there a legal definition or category that truly defines the disease and the many off spins that can occur as a result of sarcoidosis's effect on the organs. Last, but not least, as of 2008, there is no cure for sarcoidosis! There have been cases of sarcoidosis reported in virtually every organ of the body, every race, all ages, both sexes and all income brackets - worldwide. Sarcoidosis cases can be as mild as not requiring treatments and can be as extreme as causing death. Sarcoidosis is a perfect example of something that shows absolutely no prejudice and once again proves all human beings are created equal!

In my case sarcoidosis affected my lungs, liver, lymph nodes, and most importantly, my pituitary gland. Now all of a sudden my symptoms started to make sense. The only real problem I had with my lungs was I wasn't able to get enough air out. This is why I would be short of breath and cough when talking. Even the weirdness of coughing on the phone made sense because in face-to-face conversations it's okay to pause while you take a deep breath but while talking on the phone, especially in business situations, a moment of silence is an eternity, so I would try to get my sentences completed thus running out of air causing me to cough. Whew! This explained why I was short of breath while playing basketball as well.

What puzzles me is the fact my sarcoidosis started, as most cases do, on my lungs and should have showed up as an abnormality on a chest X-ray. Remember part of my routine with all seven doctors included a chest X-ray, but nothing abnormal was ever reported. The reason this bothers me so much is because when I was in the hospital, after my diagnosis in 1991, getting adjusted to my new medications they did a routine chest X-ray. This time the radiation technician saw my results and literally ran to my pulmonologist to warn him how my lungs looked and the possibility he had a terminally ill situation on his hands. I was told this by the intern who was working with my endocrinologist. Of course my pulmonologist thanked the radiation technician for his concern but he already knew what the problem was and had it under control. Personally I've never seen, nor want to see, a picture of my lungs. Now keeping in mind my symptoms started back in late 1985 and on my lungs, don't you think one of those chest X-rays showed some abnormality? Was it ignored because they didn't know what it was or did not take it seriously? It just makes me wonder how my life would be today if sarcoidosis had been detected in its early stages. After all I had been going to the doctor on a regular basis since 1986. Oh well, you can't dwell on spilled milk and dwelling on negative situations from the past over which you have no control does absolutely no good. Although it wasn't easy, with God's help and Ma-Shelle by my side I have moved on.

It was the sarcoidosis on my liver that explained the yellowing of my skin, a symptom of jaundice. The real issues, however, came from the sarcoidosis affecting my pituitary gland, therefore causing, an insufficient endocrine system or hypo pituitary, also referred to as pituitary sarcoidosis, a fairly rare form of sarcoidosis. Due to this situation there were several permanent chronic health conditions I developed and needed treatment in order to survive.

Since there's no cure for sarcoidosis, we are now partners for the rest of my life. We treat the symptoms by way of replacement medications. My endocrinologist made it a point to stress the medications we're using are in reality just replacing what my body doesn't produce on its own. The primary drug used to treat sarcoidosis in most cases, including mine, is prednisone, a commonly used steroid. Prednisone at a very high dosage was first used to put the sarcoid granulomas in remission. The damage had already been done to my organs, but at least it could be stopped from spreading. Once the sarcoidosis was in remission a reduced dosage of prednisone was given to keep it under control to prevent it from spreading once again and to help provide the steroids my body needed, but yet didn't produce naturally. Reducing prednisone is something you have to be very careful with because you just can't stop taking prednisone because it will have a dramatically negative effect on your body which could possibly be life threatening.

Prednisone can be a rough drug to tolerate. The main side effect is weight gain. I shot from about 130 pounds to about 185 pounds within a couple of weeks. You wouldn't believe the looks and uncomfortable situations I experienced with people who knew me. I tell you in America overweight people are judged and put down on a regular basis. What other group of people do you know where others can tell cruel jokes about them in public, get a good laugh and no one think twice about it - except the overweight people that is? It's sad we treat people with such disrespect and it's accepted. For me just putting on my shoes now became an ordeal.

I know a lot of people who refuse to take prednisone because of the many side effects. Unfortunately, at this point in time, prednisone is one of the primary drugs used in the treatment of sarcoidosis. I'll get into other side effects of prednisone and my other medications later in this book. At least for me I didn't experience any side effects from my medications severe enough for me to have to stop taking them. After several months I worked my way down to my daily dosage of prednisone, which I take both in the morning and at night. Additionally when other events happen in my life such as a cold, stress or anything else where my body and immune system would produce more natural steroids, I must take additional prednisone. This is a tricky situation but over the years I've learned to know when and when not to take more prednisone. I'm just thankful I'm able to tolerate the drug even if it has caused me other health problems such as weight gain, along with swollen stomach, face and eyes. Prolonged usage has been associated with other chronic health conditions such as vision problems, slow healing, and heart issues as well. At least it keeps the sarcoidosis in remission…for now.

Medication was needed for hypothyroidism as well, as a result of problems with my thyroid gland. This was what caused my skin problems, bulging eyes, mood swings and holding heat inside my body; to mention a few. Thinking back I should have recognized these symptoms because when we lived in Tallahassee Vanessa had thyroid problems for which she had surgery. She experienced the same skin, eyes, mood and heat issues as I do now, but like I've said, "When it's you that's sick your mind doesn't think logically or clearly." By the time I was experiencing these symptoms Vanessa had passed.

My body wasn't producing enough testosterone, causing me to suffer from insufficient testosterone levels, thus resulting in my male hormone problems. To combat this problem I receive an injection of depo-testosterone in my hip muscle. Since I'm scared to death of needles I go to my endocrinologist's office for them to administer the injection. We started at once a month then went to every three weeks. That turned out to not be sufficient so we went to bi-weekly, although since 2008 I'm weekly and my wife now gives me the injection at home.

As I said I'm scared to death of needles, in fact I don't even look at them. It's just something about seeing them going in that makes my skin crawl. Let me give you a tip on how you can avoid the sting of the poke when, for example, you're giving blood, something we all have to do from time to time.

When I was in the hospital my roommate was a retired pediatric dentist. He sensed I was scared of needles, since they were taking blood from me every time I turned around. My endocrinologist is one of the most detail oriented doctors around and was testing me left and right, along with monitoring my reactions to the new medications. The dentist told me the next time I'm about to be poked to blink my eyes nonstop as fast as I could and he guaranteed I wouldn't feel the poke, unless of course the nurse couldn't get my vein. When the nurse came in I tried it and sure enough I didn't feel a thing. I asked him why that technique worked and he told me when you blink your eyes that fast the brain is too busy trying to figure out if you're going to keep your eyes opened or closed to acknowledge a little poke in your body. He told me he would teach his young patients that trick to gain the confidence of the children and it worked every time. I still do the blinking trick every time I get any type of injection and it still tricks my brain every time. Give it a try.

You can treat insufficient testosterone levels with wearing a daily patch as well. I've tried this method a couple of times when my injection medication was taken off the market due to unknown problems (it was kept real secret what those problems were). For me I hated the patch, but that's just me. It was uncomfortable to wear and just bugged me.

Another method, and one I feel is the best if you can use it, is a daily gel you rub into your skin in the morning; then after a short time you can do anything you desire, like swim, sweat or shower. There was only one problem for me - my body didn't accept the medication for some unknown reason. My endocrinologist said I was the only patient he knew whose body didn't accept the medication. We tried a couple of times increasing the dosage to the maximum allowed but my body just didn't accept it. So I, as should you, just stick to what works and get my weekly injections.

The last chronic health condition I developed was diabetes insipidus. Diabetes insipidus is a rare form of diabetes (although it's not technically categorized as a diabetic disease) that causes extreme thirst and urination like no thirst or sensation you have ever experienced. My diabetes insipidus is caused by the fact my body no longer produces the hormone vasopressin, which is produced in the posterior lobe of the pituitary gland damaged by the sarcoidosis affecting that portion of my brain. The lack of this hormone causes the kidney to excrete excessive quantities of very diluted, but otherwise normal, urine. Most people only think of the kidneys in regard to urination problems but the brain, or more specifically the pituitary gland, should be considered as well. This is why the feelings I experienced regarding my thirst and having to urinate was so intense and like nothing I had felt before. It was why I had symptoms of diabetes mellitus, had problems with my teeth and a problem with producing saliva as well. All of a sudden all of those mysteries were starting to make sense!

To treat diabetes insipidus I take DDAVP, a nasal spray, twice a day. Fortunately for me, DDAVP had just recently been approved at this time; otherwise I would have required four daily injections into my kidneys. You can also get DDAVP via tablet form but like the testosterone gel my body doesn't accept the tablet. Insufficient testosterone and diabetes insipidus are two conditions you know immediately if the medications work or not, no questions about it. Always learn what works best for you and not what's best for others; and then make your decision.

Diabetes insipidus probably has the most impact on my life, although it's easily managed, because of the fact when the DDAVP stops working I immediately go into the extreme thirst and frequent urination mode. At times I'll take an additional spray to hold me over but you have to be very careful because it's just as dangerous to take too much DDAVP because your body will then retain too much fluid. Like prednisone I've learned over the years when and when not to take additional DDAVP.

After my diagnosis I placed a call to the doctor who had found something wrong with my pituitary gland and sent me to the endocrinologist, thus in my opinion, saving my life. When I got him on the phone I told him we found the source of the problem and it was sarcoidosis. I remember his response in detail as he said, "Damn!" Then after a short pause as he continued, "I'll be damn! Sarcoidosis! Gil, I don't think I ever would have gotten that one." I thanked him from the bottom of my heart for being the first doctor professional enough to have enough confidence in himself to ask for help. He simply replied, "You're welcome. After all, that's my job!"

When I was first diagnosed with sarcoidosis I think I had an initial reaction most people feel who have experienced going a long period of time getting sicker by the day and yet not getting any answers as to what was causing their health problems - relief! I was so relieved I finally had an answer to what was causing my problems! Even if I'd never heard of sarcoidosis, knew little about what a pituitary gland did, had no understanding about the chronic health conditions caused by this disease and was completely naïve about how my life was about to change, I could finally say what was wrong with me! Even if I couldn't explain the disease and people would look at me with a blank look in their eyes, at least I could say something.

The mental relief of having an answer took a tremendous weight off my shoulders. At least for the moment I was, in my mind that is, going to get back to the way my life was in 1985. I couldn't wait to start eating again, making love to the woman I loved, getting back to a full work schedule and, even more so, getting back to playing basketball. I would tell the fellows at the gym to watch out because I was coming back as a seven-foot point guard with better skills than I had before I went out. One of the most commonly known functions of the pituitary gland is controlling a person's growth, thus I was going to go from six to seven feet tall! I know, in reality I was just talking smack. As with all patients who have been diagnosed with a life altering health condition, or in my case, several life altering chronic health conditions, your life changes. Reality hit me head on in no time flat!

One of the first changes was eating. Yeah I was able to eat more but WOW. One of the side effects of prednisone is the munchies. Keep in mind I was on a high dosage of prednisone at first so I started eating everything in sight. It was weird to go to restaurants and the waiter or waitress who knew me would automatically bring a pitcher of water and pitcher of tea or pop to the table out of habit. I would think to myself, "How could I have drunk so much during a meal?" However the DDAVP now successfully controls that urge and the prednisone was making me eat, eat and eat.

One example of how this affected me was one afternoon I had just finished a big lunch of a cheeseburger and fries when Ma-Shelle called to see if I wanted to go get something to eat. I picked her up right away and we went to a local steak house where I ate from the salad bar, and not just salad but chicken wings as well, then ate my steak with fries. Of course I couldn't leave without some ice cream. I took Ma-Shelle straight home then as soon as I walked in the door (probably 45 minutes after I finished my ice cream) I put a large frozen pizza in the oven. That was when it hit me how much I was eating without even thinking about it. I had to start learning to "not" eat, something I hadn't had to do in about five years or my entire life for that matter!

As I said earlier, another side effect of prednisone is weight gain so with that side effect working on me along with eating like someone who had been stranded on a deserted island, my weight exploded. The adjustment was new and hard for me. In fact when I look at pictures of myself I actually looked like a pregnant man. In fact I still do! I hardly recognized myself! However I didn't let it stop me from trying to get into shape for my return to a busy work schedule and to the basketball court.

Unfortunately that reality hit me hard as well. I was still having trouble getting to work everyday and my energy still was not like it should be. I tried to tell myself it was the additional weight, but I think I knew it was more than that. I wasn't ready, or did not know how, to accept my new reality just yet. My body just didn't produce the energy levels as I had, even with the high dosage of prednisone. My endocrinologist once told me after a good night's sleep my energy level in the morning was about the same level as a normal person's when they go to bed after a long day.

From the time I was diagnosed in 1991 until I stopped working for EDS in 2002, I never made it into the office every day for a two weeks timeframe - not once. I know this because at first my goal was to make it every day for a month, but after a year having never come close to achieving that objective, I changed the goal to three weeks, which was also never achieved. Around 1994 the goal changed to two weeks and I still never achieved that objective either. This is something that depressed me for years because no matter how hard I tried I just couldn't accomplish this goal. In order to avoid frustration and stress we need to understand our limits so we don't make unrealistic goals for ourselves.

However some goals just seemed reachable even though after 12 years they never were. No matter how much we understand our situation, acceptance is still another story!

Chronic fatigue is one of the most depressing health conditions you can have because it makes you feel so lazy and down on yourself, even if you understand it. You can't see it or feel it. Even though your mind says do this, your body says I'm not doing that. It is a constant internal struggle that is forever changing and is something with which a patient must recognize, admit, and manage.

I was even more determined to get back to playing basketball. For me basketball was a way of life and my lifeline for socializing with other men. I had always been one of the best basketball players around and basketball kept me out of trouble or "getting beat down" on more than one occasion. If you understand the street life you know what I'm saying. I always saw myself as playing competitively until I was 40 years old and since I was only 33 years old at the time, in my mind, I had seven more years ahead of me before I retired to the slow-break leagues. After all I was now on replacement medications so I should be back to normal. Right? Wrong!

When my prednisone was reduced and I had been walking and shooting around, I knew it was time to start back against other players. I started slow with a little two on two at a goal in the park in my downtown Detroit neighborhood and won every game I played. Except for being a step slower and not having the spring I once did, I was still successful and could pretty much do what I wanted, although dunking at will was now a past memory. I was mainly a jump shooter at this time in my life anyway and once you have a pure jump shot by nature it never goes away. If you're wide open you can knock the shot down. Plus I had experience and knew all the little tricks a lot of the other players didn't quite know or if they did I was better at beating them to the punch.

My first time back at the YMCA was also successful, a curse in disguise. The other players welcomed me back and in true playground fashion, didn't take it lightly on me. Basketball is a cruel game, especially on the street, and when you're weak the predators attack. The regular ballers figured now was the time to get me back while they could for the years of abuse they had endured, but no such luck! The first day we won all three games before I was too tired and quit, on my own terms this time around, and not because I was vomiting. It felt good, I mean damn good, to have played full court basketball again, fought in competition and won. There's nothing like the satisfaction of hitting a jump shot in someone's face when there's nothing they can do about it or feeling the soreness of a good workout. It had been so long since I had felt either. I even enjoyed getting knocked around a couple of times. I couldn't wait for next week to come.

The next week during the very first game reality told me enough is enough: it is time to come down to earth! I was bringing the ball down court. I stopped at the top of the key, faked left then pushed right to pull up for a jumper. Instead of pulling up I heard a loud popping sound; it felt as someone had stepped on my ankle and I went down. I looked around quickly to see who had stepped on me or if a ball had rolled out on the court since sometimes players on the sideline will shoot a quick jumper at the other goal while the ball is in play on the other end of the court. However, all I saw was the man guarding me laying the ball up at the other goal. I didn't know what had happened but I did know something wasn't right.

I was able to walk but not move my ankle and I wasn't in any real pain. I was even able to drive myself home, as it was my left ankle that was hurt. After a few hours I went to the emergency room and found out I had ripped my Achilles tendon almost completely through. I was put in a cast for eight weeks. On my next visit to my endocrinologist the following week I received the dose of reality that made me finally understand it was time for me to learn to live with my new health conditions because my life had changed forever. I didn't have certain daily luxuries other individuals had anymore, and I better learn how to live within my new reality successfully because I was never going to be the way I was in 1985. I remember his first words to me, in a stern tone like a parent chastising his/her child, "Who told you to play full court basketball? Not me!"

At this point I began a mental adjustment, as I knew my health was going to dictate my life from now on. I started to think about my life and what did I do to deserve having my life changed this way? To come to grips with the reality that my life would forever be changing could have driven me crazy with self-pity - if I had let it.

After a few weeks of depression and self-pity I told myself I wasn't going to let my new health conditions keep me from living a fulfilling life. Life has too much to offer to stop living just because I could no longer do the things I once did. Truth is we all experience change in our lives as we get older. It's just when you have a chronic health condition it's more sudden and obvious. So what if I couldn't play basketball anymore, I could still watch it. Now I could use my time for other interest like enjoying walks and spending time doing other activities of interest with my family and friends. I started to adjust my life by trying to understand what I could and couldn't do successfully. "Can't" wasn't such a bad word anymore. Instead I had learned to accept in a positive way my new life style.

This was the hardest thing I had to do, and still is, as I have to look at myself everyday because my health is ever changing. To help with my new reality the one thing I did was get out of management, even though I loved it and was good at it. It was unfair for me not to be in the office everyday because as a manager, personnel issues are part of the job and I felt it was my responsibility to physically be in the office and available to my staff. I tried but this was not something I could do so the decision had to be made to find another position for which I could be just as productive for the corporation, and in addition, could work from home when needed. Therefore I talked to my manager honestly and in turn became a Business Analyst and managed projects, not people. This way I could have conference calls and work on the system or project from my home, while still being productive for EDS and adjusted my work methods to be open with everyone I worked with about my health. I kept very organized notes or folders so anyone could look at them and understand where we were in the scope of the project or what needed to be done along with making copies of them for me to take home. As a result of understanding and learning how to work with the reality of my new health conditions now everyone involved was able to work together. It was extra work for me but it allowed me to be successful from a business and health perspective, a win-win situation for my co-workers, management, our customers and me. I continued doing this until my health finally got the best of me and I left the corporate world in 2002.

My life has continuously changed since 1991, causing me to stay on top of my situation, although mentally I do have my lapses. My chronic health conditions have also increased. Since 1991 I've developed hypertension, an irregular heartbeat, severe acid reflux, high cholesterol, sleep apnea, damaged nerve endings, swollen eyes, face and stomach from continued use of prednisone, cataracts in both eyes, blurred vision, became anemic, and developed diabetes mellitus…to go along with my insufficient endocrine system, hypothyroidism, insufficient testosterone levels, severe muscle cramps, chronic fatigue and diabetes insipidus. In 2009 I'm taking approximately 17 pills, 4 nasal sprays and sleep with a Continuous Positive Airway Pressure (CPAP) machine on a daily basis, along with getting a bi-weekly injection and constantly checking my blood sugar levels. In February 2006 (one day before my 48th birthday) I was given my last chance of medication adjustments, a stern lecture to walk everyday and control my diet more efficiently in order to attempt to keep my sugar levels under control. Unfortunately it didn't work; therefore insulin has become a normal routine in my life, and for someone who hates needles as much as I do, well let's just say the phase, "Do what you have to do!" is once again part of my daily vocabulary.

Change is something we all must learn to accept and deal with in everyday situations, but when you're a patient with health conditions that affect your everyday life you have to be even more alert and aware of your situation. Learning to adapt to change now becomes a survival skill as opposed to just going with the flow. Your quality of life not only depends on learning to successfully notice, accept, then adapt to change, but being aware of it on a regular basis as well. Like any profession you learn how to be a "Professional Patient".

The physical aspects are actually the easiest part of the puzzle. It's easier to deal with something physical because you can see or feel it, giving you a sense of reality with what you're dealing. You know you can't jump up and down if your leg is broken because that's a physical fact, but it's a different ball game when you want to do something but your body is experiencing chronic fatigue and for some reason you just can't get going.

The mental aspect is what's the most difficult, or maybe better put…your everyday physiological warfare of living with your health situation and the impact it has not only on your life but those around you as well. Physiological warfare might sound a bit dramatic to some but the reality is when you deal with life, as a patient with a chronic health disease, everyday is a battle and in order to win the war with your disease or diseases you must win the majority of the battles. War is about life and death, and just as a soldier does all he/she can to survive, you as a patient must do the same because anytime you fight a disease, especially on a chronic basis, your survival is at stake. You are your own commander in chief, general and soldier! Therefore the most important thing you as a patient must learn in order to be successful in maintaining your quality of life is what's the best strategy for you to win the mental battles you'll face in all aspects of being a patient.

This is a question only you can answer because each of us reacts and thinks differently in regard as how to handle our health issues, especially from a mental aspect. What we all must do in order to figure out our best strategy is first, like understanding our body, we must look deep into our souls and come to grips with the reality of our situation. This is extremely difficult to do but must be done. You see our health, especially in today's world, involves more than just dealing with the physical aspects of our situation. There's the financial burdens being sick can bring such as: paying medical bills, missing work and not receiving normal income thus being dependent on others for income. There's the guilt we might feel for the additional burdens placed on our loved ones, especially if you're an individual who has always been in total control of his/her situation.

In my case it has taken a lot of years of internal struggles to come to grips with the reality of my health situation, and to be honest, I still struggle on a daily basis. Even though I believe I have a very good understanding of how sarcoidosis and the other chronic health conditions affect me physically, mentally it is still a challenge. As a human being and a man, I don't want to give up some of the things I have done or feel I should be doing in order to support myself and my family. However the reality is, I can't, and that's a harder pill to swallow than any medication I've been prescribed.

Everyday you're forced to look yourself in the mirror and accept your conditions. You have to continue to force yourself not to give in to feeling sorry for yourself and blaming the world for your situation. It's critical to remember your health doesn't define who you are - you do!

This is true regardless of your health situation, or any other situation. It's your attitude and ability to face your reality in a positive fashion that makes you who you are as a human being. It might be easier to just quit, in fact quitting is without a doubt the easy way out in anything you do. However, when it comes to living with chronic health conditions, quitting could have dramatic effects on your quality of life, on those around you or on life itself. So you must mentally accept quitting is not an option! It is of great importance for you to understand your situation, to accept it and then to learn how to deal with it mentally or else. None of us want to experience the "or else"!

Over the years I've had to accept my inability to work a "regular" job and understand when I felt I could or couldn't perform required duties without hurting myself or whatever business at which I was attempting to be successful. I had to make some soul searching tough decisions. I've had to learn when I was physically, or mentally, able to attend family or personal events and not cause myself to get sick from doing something I had no business doing, but really wanted to do. You hope loved ones will understand and if they truly love you unconditionally and you've been honest with them, they will. On the other hand I've had to learn to face the reality everyone doesn't understand how I feel, how my health affects my life or my wife's life as well, even those close to me. When looking at me you can't tell anything is seriously wrong; it's not something that's obvious. Even if you're aware of my health condition and you aren't around me on a daily basis, you tend to forget. This is normal and something I understand. As a result I've had to dig deep in my soul and learn how to put all of the negative vibes aside so I can deal with my life in a positive manner, regardless of what others, even loved ones, might think. Once you understand how you feel and how your body will function from a physical and mental aspect, then that is when you have truly learned how to be a patient and you are in control of your own life. Of course the next day everything changes once again!

You can't get comfortable mentally with your situation to the point you stop being aware of the changes you experience both physically and mentally because your health changes on a regular basis. Just based on the fact you grow older each day causes a healthy body to change. The hard part is in today's environment as a patient it is not only your health you have to keep on top of, but also the processes of your insurance, new doctor procedures, family issues and a multitude of other factors your health situation affects. If you are too sick or mentally drained to take care of your situation, it is a must that you have someone who can step in for you when needed. That someone must be aware of vital information such as your health problems, including doctors and medications, your insurance and financial obligations. It is the patient's responsibility to ensure that the situation is taken care of by being prepared for any circumstance or event that might occur - beforehand! We must all be responsible for ourselves. After all, it's you, the patient, that's going to feel the consequence of your actions or non-actions. Learn and keep on learning what it takes to be a successful patient!

...2...

Life is a daily evolution. Regardless of what negative changes you experience in life remember life is not always fair. However you are always in control of how you accept your fate and in turn make any negative situation in your life a positive motivation. You are responsible for your own life!

3
Learning How To Be A Successful Patient

Learning how to be a successful patient can be tricky. This might sound silly or too simple but learning how to be a patient in the 21st century is the most important step in getting the best medical care needed for your situation, be you a patient living with chronic health conditions or just the patient in good health that's forced to visit the doctor from time to time. You must always remember "It's your health at stake thus you are responsible for the success you have."

To start let's get an understanding of what the word "patient" means literally and what it means in reality. The word "patient" has a Latin root meaning "suffering". When we look in Webster's Tenth Edition Collegiate Dictionary a couple of definitions read (1) *Bearing pains or trials calmly or without complaint*; (2) *An individual awaiting or under medical care and treatment*. Another word associated with the word patient is "patience", defined as (1) *The capacity, habit, or fact of being patient*. Literally these words go hand in hand and these definitions are suitable. However let's look at the reality of today's medical environment and define "patient" as you must learn to understand it.

For the modern patient the word would better be defined as (1) *Learn how to wait without adding the burden of stress by being prepared to wait because it is what you will be doing the majority of your time*! Regardless of what you do in the medical environment be prepared to wait. It's unfortunate, because that's just how it is at this time. Learn to be prepared because if you're prepared, it will probably still bother you, but at least it won't be unexpected and your stress level shouldn't be as intense.

The logic reminds me of those people who get up before dawn on the Friday after Thanksgiving to get the so-called first Holiday sales. I know about this because Ma-Shelle and I do it as well. We're not looking for sales because nowadays the first Holiday sales realistically start in July. For us it's tradition and the best time to people watch. The one thing everyone can guarantee to experience during the mad Friday is you're going to have to wait in long lines no matter what you try to do. There's no getting around it. So why do individuals get so frustrated when they have to wait, to the point their stress levels go through the roof and they end up having a miserable time? They knew ahead of time they weren't going to be the only people in the stores, in restaurants or on the road but yet some folks look so surprised at the long lines. Understanding you're going to have to wait gets you in the frame of mind that you must be patient all day. Once you understand this fact and accept there's nothing you can do about it, you will enjoy the experience.

The same holds true for being a patient in today's medical environment. Understand you're going to have to wait. Be prepared mentally and your experience will not be as stressful as it would if you get yourself all worked up because you have to wait. I know this can be difficult when you're sick but this is something you need to achieve successful patient status. You must understand and come to grips with waiting because changing this fact is out of your control. Don't worry about those things you can't control and change what you can control. Because this is one of those situations out of your control, learn to deal with it.

Hopefully things will get better in the future and hopefully you will luck out at certain doctor appointments. For example, I've never had to wait more than five minutes at my sleep specialist for an appointment, even when I had to update my records. As long as medical professionals double and triple book appointments or don't schedule ample time for each patient visit this will be a problem. Just like airlines overbook flights, a lot of doctors do the same and it's just physically impossible to see two patients at the same time. Someone is going to have to wait past his/her appointment time.

I guess, from a personal perspective, what bugs me about this attitude is the patient's time is just as important as the doctor's, especially when you factor in the fact that the patient isn't feeling well. If other businesses can keep appointments and schedules, there's no reason why a medical professional can't either, except when an emergency occurs or a patient has an unexpected situation that causes the doctor to be behind. Until we get more considerate doctors, a sufficient number of quality nurses, prevention of insurance company's pressure, solution to the current health care coverage crisis we are currently experiencing in America, and a change in the overall cultural attitude of certain, not all, medical professionals that the needs and rights of the patient should come first, we, as patient, must accept that waiting will always be a fact of our medical life. Hence, we, as patients, have to learn personally the best way to deal with waiting.

Trust me, getting an attitude with the medical assistances or nurses will not, and I repeat, **will not**, get you in any faster or get you any better service. They're human as well and are probably just as frustrated with being overworked as you are with having to wait. We'll deal with relationships later in this book but for now understand that relationships are a two way street and you must build a positive relationship with your medical professionals in order to be successful. Getting frustrated at the ones who will eventually call you back is not how to build positive relationships nor does it do you any good.

Let me tell you a little story about my father to emphasize how learning the process of waiting will eliminate or reduce your stress level. My father was diagnosed with lung cancer in May 2004. A little background on him includes that he lived in Perry, a rural North Florida town, having moved there from Tennessee in 1953. He was a popular high school teacher, baseball/football coach, softball umpire, and most importantly, a very successful varsity basketball coach until the late-1970s, retiring from the school system in 1988. When you hung out with him almost everyone we saw he had either taught or coached, and most likely their children as well. Golfing was another favorite activity; in fact today he's an honorary member of the country club and has had a tournament in his honor. He was well known by all of the golfers in the area, not to mention the fact he lived in a small town "where everyone knows your name". In other words he was accustomed to everyone knowing him and usually making a fuss over him. You know the saying, "A big fish in a small pond and perfectly content." That was my father.

He had never been sick to amount to anything in his life so when he was diagnosed with cancer it blew his mind and made for a tremendous adjustment, both physically and mentally. Once he was diagnosed I immediately flew from Detroit not only to take him to his radiation treatments, which were an hour's drive each way, but also to help him and my mother, with all of the other factors involved with his being sick such as insurance issues and getting his prescription drugs from his doctors since he had no drug coverage. But primarily he had to learn the process of being a patient, because for him, he was entering a foreign but essential world.

He honestly expected for everyone to give him priority, and he expected to be able to walk into any doctor's office at any time and be seen right away like it was 1960. When we're sick, especially when we have a disease we know can take our life, everyone feels they're the only and most important patient their doctor has. In reality we really are one in many because a quality doctor will give each patient equal attention and care.

It was so frustrating for him to have to wait, sometimes for quite a while, for an appointment. He would complain loudly to anyone who would listen and tell me he was going to walk back and see the doctor, and he honestly thought he could, after all...he was Coach Barr. Lord knows, don't let someone who came in after him get called in before him. "I was here before them! Why do they get called before me? I'm going home!" he would bark out at no one in particular while fidgeting in his seat. I would try to explain to him there are several doctors and specialists in the office (in rural areas a lot of tests are conducted on certain days by physicians from other areas) and not everyone was here for the same reason or to see the same doctor. However my words went in one ear and out the other as his impatience and stress levels grew with every passing moment, even if it had only been five or ten minutes past his appointment time. You can only imagine how he was after 30 minutes of wait time!

Let's not forget the endless forms to fill out. He would again complain loudly when asked to fill out a form and usually didn't have the necessary information on him. When he would go to another doctor or have a test performed and was asked to fill out their paperwork, he would protest loudly and rudely. I would once again calmly explain this doctor is different from his doctor at home and they too needed his personal information. "Well I've already filled this junk out more than once!" he would snap back. I tell you, it could be down right embarrassing at times, but what can you do? Fortunately most of the staff he interacted with seemed to understand and was for the most part responsive to the best of their ability. Plus there's a noticeable difference, in a positive manner, in the way cancer patients are treated. But still! Things would be a lot easier and less stressful once he learned the process and understood what it took to be a successful patient.

To make a long story short, he tried and eventually, although still impatient, learned the process and what to expect, thus being prepared for the experience. There were two situations that showed me he had finally accepted the fact he was inevitably a patient and had learned what it took to be successful and ease the stress you feel when you're sick, getting ready for surgery or going through a specific treatment process.

The first came in February 2005. He was scheduled to have his coronary artery cleaned out, as it was about 90% clogged. When we arrived for his surgery we went through the administrative process. However, this time when he approached the station and was given the clipboard of paperwork, he took it without complaint, taking out his insurance cards and notebook with his other vital information and went right to work. In a few minutes he was finished, gave the completed, yes completed, documents to the staff member and was called back in no time flat. What a difference understanding what would be required and being prepared made! He had learned complaining wasn't going to make the paperwork go away so instead he was prepared. The stress level and hassle was now at a minimum and you could see it in his eyes.

The second time came in May 2005. He had been diagnosed with cancer for the second time, this time in his bladder and had started radiation treatments again. This time around, due to some health issues of my own, I wasn't able to come down until after the first week of treatments had been completed. He had told me on about the fourth day he was going to go earlier because one of the machines was being repaired. When I gave him my daily call to see how his day went he was in a jolly mood. I asked him how the treatment went and he laughed and said, "I had to wait about 40 minutes but I already knew one of the machines was down. When they called me back I joked with the volunteer that I was just getting ready to come inform her I had been waiting more than 30 minutes (there's a sign that says if you've been waiting more than 30 minutes for your appointment to let someone know). Of course I already knew I was going to have to wait since they only had one machine and told her I was just joking, but we still all got a kick out of it!" We laughed and I told him, "Daddy, you now understand one of the tricks as to what it takes to be a successful patient." I could only imagine the fit he would have thrown a year ago when he was first diagnosed!

Of course as the saying goes, "You can't teach an old dog new tricks." He still had his moments, especially when he became sicker and his hope that he was going to get his normal life back started to diminish. Even then, after he had his moments, he would comment he knew he was wrong and he needed to be more patient. I would tell him how proud I was of him and his ability to accept the changes taking place in his life. The fact is we are all human and even if we understand the concept of being patient, we are still sick and in the case of a life-ending condition, scared. Although it's a first step to understand this fact of a patient's life, it can still be frustrating, that's just human nature. As simple as it sounds and as hard as it is to do, I promise learning to wait patiently will help relieve the stress levels, and thus, make your medical visit go smoother and more successful. I can honestly say I am so proud of how my father adjusted to his terminal health situation!

Another step for success is to learn and understand the processes and procedures in today's medical environment. This knowledge will, without a doubt, not only ease your stress level, but will enable you to get the treatments in a timelier manner as well. Aside from learning how you can pass the time of waiting without stressing yourself out too much, there are many other areas you, as a patient or caregiver, must learn and understand in order to achieve ultimate success. Some of those areas include, (1) learning the insurance process, especially in the HMO environment, (2) understanding the processes of the many doctors and specialists you'll be required to see and for what each is responsible, (3) learning where you can find the least expensive yet quality prescription medications you need, and, most of all, (4) building positive relationships with the many medical professional you will encounter.

As always, let's be upfront. Learning and understanding the processes required of today's medical patients will be frustrating at times, to say the least. Each office or facility does things just a little bit differently and everyone you deal with is a unique individual with a unique personality. Therefore always ask as many questions as you need to in order to understand what you're responsible for and the best way each office's process works. Never assume what you did at your last doctor is what they do here. Even making appointments can be tricky at times. Miscommunications is a major problem, as there have been times when the patient is waiting on the doctor's office to call, while the doctor's office is waiting for the patient to make the follow-up or test appointment. The result is usually the patient going longer than he/she should before the follow-up or test is scheduled, which could have a dramatic effect or cause more in depth treatments having to be performed.

This happened to me when I first went on my high dosage of prednisone. When I was released from the hospital I thought when I had my follow-up appointment with my endocrinologist he would reduce my high dosage of prednisone based on how I was doing. When I went to my appointment the first thing he said to me was, "My you have put on a lot of weight! What dosage of prednisone does the pulmonologist have you on?" Oops…my mistake! I should have made a follow-up appointment with the pulmonologist to check the progress of the prednisone in regard to putting the sarcoidosis in remission on my lungs but I was under the impression my endocrinologist was responsible for that. I may have been dealing with the medical profession on a regular basis for over five years, but I still didn't have a good grasp on who did what, resulting in a major miscommunication. As a result of my misunderstanding of the process and instructions when I was released from the hospital (I was just wanting to get out of there!), I spent a few weeks longer than I should have on the very high dosage of prednisone. In the end it turned out no harm was done. I was lucky! However that experience taught me to always ask and make sure I understand who's calling whom to make appointments.

Timeliness can have a major impact on the seriousness of a condition or how much treatment will be needed. I can't emphasize enough the importance of early detection of any health condition, and miscommunications or not understanding the processes can lead to life altering delays. I have no doubt if I had known what I know now in regard to how to advocate for myself and how the medical environment processes worked, it wouldn't have taken over five years to diagnose me with sarcoidosis, and without a doubt, I wouldn't have the multiple chronic health conditions I live with today!

In addition you must understand what needs to take place from an insurance standpoint. If you have an HMO and need a referral it's the patient's responsibility to ensure the referral is available at the specialist. Timing is everything. Most doctor's offices require a minimum of anywhere from three to seven business days to provide a referral, except for emergency situations. Having the referral or a method of payment, either by another type of insurance or cash, will determine if and when your test or service will be performed. In fact some specialists don't need referrals anymore but will require a letter from your primary doctor giving them permission to see you. I know because I was just blindsided by this process! Don't allow your misunderstanding of the processes to delay your necessary treatments, as just an additional week could have a lifetime affect on your quality of life.

Don't be naive and think you can get your appointment or test done even if you don't have the required paperwork or method of payments. I've seen more times than not the rule is, if you don't have your referral or method of payment you don't receive the service until you do. After all, the medical profession is a business and you can't go to the grocery store and leave with food unless you pay the cashier first, nor can you expect them to let you slide and take the chance of eating the cost of their service. Understand what you need to do beforehand and do it! I will discuss in more detail later in this book what you can do to achieve these understandings from an insurance standpoint; for now just comprehend that you, the patient, must learn what needs to take place in order to receive proper medical treatment and successful results regarding the processes of both the medical professionals and your insurance coverage in order that your health not suffer unnecessarily.

Another vital area of importance you, as a patient, must learn to do is understand and listen to your own body. Your body will give you signs and warnings when things are starting to go wrong. There are several red flags when it comes to understanding your body signs. Some obvious ones are lack of energy, loss of appetite, loss of weight, mood swings, not wanting to do the things you normally enjoy, avoiding other people, changing restroom habits (either urinating, diarrhea or constipation), retiring or waking up at a different time, and just plain old feeling bad.

Pain is probably the most obvious sign. Learn the not so obvious signs as well, because they could be more important and informative than the obvious. Usually by the time pain kicks in you have a problem, but other signs, when acted upon, can possibly allow the issue to be treated before pain or more serious issues begin. Any changes in your overall health should be a warning sign to mention to your medical professional.

One such subtle sign is your body odor. If you start having a different body odor, it could be your body telling you something is wrong. As an example, if you have a bad tooth you'll start to experience bad breath; your body will produce a different body odor if something is going on that shouldn't be. Don't down play the change especially if you're taking care of your body grooming in the same manner as you always have. As a caregiver it's also important, although awkward, to address any changes you notice in body odor since you're around the patient or loved one. Because you get used to your own body odor and don't really notice the change, it might take a loved one or caregiver to be brutally honest with you. Listen with an open mind and without attitude! Regardless of the source, understanding changes in body odor can be an early detection sign and possibly life saving occurrence. Learn to be aware with an open mind!

Experiencing slight pains in your arms could indicate maybe a stroke is on the way or a slight chest pain might not be heartburn but a warning to get your blood pressure checked. Pain in your legs could indicate maybe your arteries are getting clogged or yellowing of your skin, as was one of my symptoms, could indicate some type of liver problem. Learn to recognize when changes occur with your body, and, most importantly, learn to listen to them and tell your doctor immediately. God made the human body to survive and do all it can to warn you when something is wrong. Only you truly know how you feel and only you can truly articulate those feelings.

Doctors are intelligent people but no one can read your mind. Don't expect any medical professional to be able to diagnose what's wrong with you if you don't tell them exactly how you feel. When you take your car to the shop you make sure you tell the mechanic all of the knocks your engine has been making, then shouldn't you tell your doctor all of the unusual changes to your body? If you don't make your mechanic guess what's wrong with your car, don't make your doctor guess what's wrong with your body. You can always get another car but your body is the only one available to you.

You must learn to understand what you feel and remember any sign could mean something only your doctor will recognize. The importance of learning to understand and listen to your own body is one of the most critical factors of being a successful patient, or to put it more bluntly, it is one of the most important factors in ensuring your quality of life, or for that matter, life itself. Learn to understand and listen well. Even more importantly - react.

There's still more to learning how to be a patient than just learning to be patient, learning the processes or learning to understand and listen to your own body. There's learning how to deal with the physical and mental aspects of being sick, as they both intertwine and are ever changing. Just like learning about life is an ongoing experience, as the saying goes, "You learn something new everyday". Learning about your health and how to deal with it successfully is an everyday learning experience as well. Whether you're living with chronic health conditions, have been diagnosed with an immediate life threatening disease, have had a life altering experience that changed your health condition or are just dealing with a temporary, but still life altering, situation such as a bad case of the flu, the mental aspects and changes you'll experience, must be understood and dealt with in a positive manner.

Keeping a positive mental frame of mind and approach to your changing health condition is critical in the successful results you obtain. Even just growing old causes physical changes you must learn to deal with from a mental aspect. Trust me, as I speak from personal experience. There is nothing more dramatic from a mental perspective than having your life changed due to your physical health changing, even if you know why the changes are taking place. Dealing with the ongoing physical and mental stress is an everyday challenge and each of us handles it in a different manner. You must learn what's best for you!

As a successful patient one of the most fundamental duties you must perform is learning when to advocate for your rights. As a patient you can't depend on others to get it right for you; you must ensure they get it right because, worth stressing again, it's your health and quality of life at stake, not theirs. There are so many areas needing your attention such as the doctors you see, the success of appointments, the treatment of your doctors and staff, remembering to inform your doctor of all problems and reactions to treatments, insurance benefits, medication costs, and probably the most frequent area, billing. This is a lot for which to deal, especially when the physical and mental stresses of your condition can have a major impact on your ability to handle all of these other issues or you've not yet learned how to be a patient in the 21st century. However the reality is…you have to! This is another reason why eliminating as much stress as possible by learning what we've discussed thus far, is so important to your overall success as a patient. Your responsibilities as a patient never stop!

There are two basic but extremely important things you must learn, in order not to overdo yourself or waste time and energy on issues that are either out of your control or not worth fighting in regard to issues pertaining to billing or other areas where you're entitled to something you didn't receive in the correct manner, or to your satisfaction. The first thing is to learn "when" to advocate an issue. There are some issues that are either not worth the time and effort you'll spend on them or you just aren't going to win. These are times you have to look at your own principles and determine if the issue is important enough for you to advocate for, even if you feel you will lose, it might be worth calling attention to for the next time.

An example could include being overcharged for an office visit or procedure performed on you. If the amount is small, let's say $10, a lot of people will just pay the $10 instead of going through what could be a long, intimidating process to get it corrected. I hope you aren't one of those people because being overcharged for any amount is wrong. Look at it like this…if a doctor or facility overcharges 200,000 patients $10 and only 100,000 challenge them while the other 100,000 pays the $10 then someone just made $1,000,000 unjustly. That's no different from robbing the bank of $1,000,000, which is a felony.

Personally, I'll fight a $5 overcharge if I have to, just for principle alone, although I must admit there have been a very few times I just didn't have the energy or my frustration levels were so high I just let it slide. I felt bad about not fighting it but the amount didn't hurt me financially and the time and effort I would have spent fighting it would have just done more damage healthwise at the time, consequently, I had to live with a decision with which I disagreed. Reality can sometimes be hard and unfair but it is what it is!

There are times when you're charged for visits or procedures that you never had or your insurance company or Medicare were charged. Are they worth the energy and effort? I hope so! Patients will receive Explanations Of Benefits (EOB) in the mail explaining everything billed to your insurance. A lot of times the "patient amount owed" will be $0, yet there will be items wrongfully billed to your insurance policy. Most patients just look at the "patient amount owed" and if it's $0 they either don't look at the detail or don't worry about it. It's human nature, but, in reality, this hurts us all because in the end insurance premiums for all of us will be raised. It's always the patient or consumer who pays the bill when services rise. Have you ever heard of any business not passing on costs to their customers or cutting services, when losing money?

Once I received a bill for a hospital stay that had a lot of services wrongfully billed. Now I didn't owe anything because my hospital stay was covered 100% but the facility was billing my insurance policy approximately $1,000 for services I didn't receive. I called the hospital and insurance company to let them know of the mistake. By the time I talked to everyone I had probably spent an hour of my time. An audit was conducted and in about a month I received a call from the hospital informing me I was right and the charges had been deleted. In the end I still didn't have to pay anything but I saved my insurance company over a $1,000 and hopefully helped keep our rates down for a while. The point is I felt it was worth my time to correct this issue even though there was nothing in it for me…directly. You too have to determine when issues are worth fighting with your time and effort.

Another area is customer service and results. Lord knows, I wish I had known how to advocate for myself when I kept going to the same doctor for so long while getting no results nor knowing how to demand I be sent to a specialist. I can't even imagine how much better my health and quality of life would be today or how much suffering I would have avoided if I had only known when and how to inquire for myself. I'm not bitter anymore and actually take some responsibility for my inability to be correctly diagnosed because I just kept going back for more of the same until God led me to the chiropractor. We as patients must have the frame of mind like with any service, we're customers, only with our health at stake. If you aren't getting the service or results you think are worth your business you must act, without intimidation or hesitation.

We, as patients, must understand the medical environment is a business and the bottom line of any business, regardless of what self-righteous hype or propaganda they might tell you, is to make money. It's just like the reality that everyone who works, regardless of what he/she tells you, works for money. The only groups of people who don't are those who volunteer without pay or donate their complete salary to charity. The next time someone tells you they don't work for money, ask them to donate their entire salary to sarcoidosis research or the American Cancer Society. If they say anything except yes then immediately do it, they work for money. Money might not be a priority for some but they wouldn't work the same job without it. The same is true for your doctor, pharmacy, and medical facilities. Understanding and remembering this fact enables you, the patient/customer, to use the ultimate power in your control, your money or consumer power. I promise you if you don't get the results you desire, then take your business elsewhere and urge others to do the same, that specific doctor, pharmacy or medical facility will either change their ways or go out of business. The only difference with the medical business is their customers are usually feeling bad, not in the proper frame of mind and our culture doesn't look at medical services the same as other businesses such as let's say retail. However the business bottom line is the same for both - make a profit. So I guess a lot of times it's our own fault or should I say, if we must blame someone else, it is the fault of our cultural programming.

It's hard to honestly look at yourself and your health situation, especially when all you want is to feel better. However the reality is we must first tell our doctors everything wrong with us every time we talk to them, and we must understand if a treatment isn't working for us, we're not going to get better. This is our responsibility as a patient. Learning when to aggressively demand what's important can make a tremendous difference in your quality of life, both now and in the future.

Don't be intimidated because it's a medical professional with which you're dealing or don't let the myth or mystique that can be instilled in your mind that they have a better understanding than you cause you not to act on your own best interest. No one knows your body and situation better than you. Even more importantly, don't be intimidated by someone who acts like he/she knows what he/she is doing when deep down you know or strongly believe you're right. If you don't fight for your rights, who will?

The second thing you must learn is "how" to speak up for yourself. Understanding processes and who can make decisions will save you so much time and frustrations I can't even begin to describe. Again look at other businesses. If you're getting bad service in a restaurant or retail store, you don't waste your time trying to get satisfaction from the server or clerk. No, you ask to speak to the manager and if that doesn't work you get the address or number for the district manager and so on until you get a satisfactory solution or take your business elsewhere. As a patient you must do the same.

If you have billing issues learn to whom to take the issue that will get you results instead of going on and on with a clerk who just gives you the runaround. If they tell you they'll get you an answer in a certain timeframe, give them an opportunity, but if they don't keep their word or give you a status as to why not, don't hesitate going to the next level. Understand the appeal process if you get a result with which you don't agree and if you don't understand the process, ask until you do. Have the facility or insurance company send you the process in writing because as a patient you have the prerogative to receive your rights in writing.

Following the correct processes will save you time, money and effort because when you do it the right way you put the burden on the provider to address the problem. Never be afraid to take it to another level if you aren't getting satisfaction or you feel bad because you think you might be getting someone in trouble. Maybe they just don't have the authority to make a decision so cut out the middle person. If they aren't doing their job then you're saving the next person the aggravation. That's part of management's job to ensure customers are satisfied,

and again, as a patient, you're the customer of your medical professional and insurance company because without your business they have
no business. Remember that fact and use your power as a consumer effectively! Learn "when" and "how" to advocate for your rights. It's your
personal duty.

Learning to be a successful patient takes a lot of effort at times
while sometimes just good old experience helps you be successful.
Learning to be a patient is the first step to having successful results
regarding your health care from both a physical, mental and financial
standpoint. Once you have successfully learned what it takes to be a
successful patient then the real journey begins!

...3...

**Patience is a virtue we all must learn in order to relieve unnecessary
stresses in our lives, especially in the medical environment. We are
responsible for our own frame of mind and how we personally deal
with life's situations. Don't let things out of your control have a negative effect on your life and for those negative things for which you have
control…change them immediately!**

4
3-Step Philosophy For Success

It took me years before I started to understand how to deal with my drastic change in health and accept the fact sarcoidosis, and the related chronic health conditions, were my partners for life. My primary strategy was learning from my mistakes and trust in my inner voice. When you have never been sick to amount to anything then all of a sudden your health dictates your every move, it's a trial and error daily routine to find how to be successful and live a productive life.

I went through a lot of depression, without confiding in anyone, and experienced many false hopes. When I would have successes it seemed those successful events were just followed by more false realities and depression. I went through all of the self-pity moods then the "I can conquer the world" mentalities until at the end of the day I was just confused. There had to be a better process for successfully living with these chronic health conditions!

I was trying to work a full 40 hour week but couldn't. I would get very depressed then I would make it into the office for a week or so and start to think finally I'm back to normal. Then one of those days would hit me from nowhere. I kept thinking I could still play basketball and might play a good game of H.O.R.S.E. then decided to try a little two on two. I would end up paying for it for the next week, again falling back into a state of depression. It seemed every time I had something planned my body would shut me down.

After about three or four years into my sarcoidosis life, I decided the best way, or for me the only way, to live with my health situation and still be happy, was my "3-Step Philosophy". Here's how it works.

Step-1…Learn all you can and get a good understanding of your health situation!

There are several ways you can accomplish this step. One is to talk to your doctor openly and ask any questions regarding how your health condition and medications "should" affect you. You must keep in mind the word "should" because each of us is unique and just because something is supposed to affect you a certain way doesn't mean it will. Be careful not to predetermine how you are going to feel but instead be aware of what might occur and let your doctor know the results. This is extremely important with your medications because we all react to the same medications differently.

Your primary doctor is not the only medical professional whom you can discuss how you should feel or learn about your conditions or medications. Request to speak with a specialist such as a dietician or someone who is an expert in your health conditions field (*ie*: a doctor who specializes in treating sarcoidosis or diabetes patients). Your pharmacist is a good resource to discuss the history of the medications you take. Just keep in mind your doctor is your primary source of advice because he/she knows your history, which another expert will not have. When it comes to your health every detail makes a difference and no question is a bad one.

Another method of learning about your health conditions or medications is to do research yourself. In our modern world the Internet is a powerful learning tool that anyone can access. Information is available on almost every subject and is growing by the day. To start your research all you need to do is go to any search engine, such as Google. com or Yahoo.com, and enter a keyword like the name of your health condition or medication, then press the "enter" key. You will receive a list of web sites that contain your keyword and from there you can choose which web site you want to view. When I first started trying to learn about sarcoidosis and gather information on the Internet I would enter the keyword "sarcoidosis" and only a few links would pop up. Today there are thousands.

The Internet is available 24 hours a day and available to anyone worldwide, as long as you have an Internet connection available. It's an excellent resource to communicate with other patients as well. I'm a strong believer when it comes to getting advice on how to cope with a health condition, side effect, the mental stresses or the effect your health conditions can have on your overall life, there is no better resource than another patient who is experiencing the same as you.

Communicating with someone who can personally relate to what you feel is priceless. It doesn't matter that my wife spends her life with me and sees what I go through, unless she experiences it herself she can't truly understand. My endocrinologist has treated sarcoidosis and diabetes patients for years, and is excellent, but he still can't truly understand how we feel if he doesn't experience it. Psychologists can have years of training and experience talking to patients dealing with the mental pressures of living with chronic health conditions but they can't truly understand how a person feels mentally unless they live with those chronic health conditions on a daily basis themselves.

I went years without ever even meeting a person with diabetes insipidus. I viewed the Diabetes Insipidus Foundation's web site on a regular basis. I read other patient stories and even wrote an article for their newsletter and web site, but I never physically talked to anyone. In August 2004 I spoke at their first annual conference in Baltimore and for the first time in my life I could look at the audience when I described the unique feelings of intense thirst and frequent urination and know the nods I was receiving from those in attendance were genuine because they experienced it as well. I can't describe the feeling of finally seeing firsthand I wasn't the only person in the world who had diabetes insipidus and what I felt as a result, both from a physical and mental perspective, was shared by others.

Other health conditions are no different. To be able to communicate in person, on the phone, via e-mail or via an online support group to others with sarcoidosis is something no one without the disease can provide regardless of how much they understand you or the basis of the condition. To talk to someone who takes prednisone daily as you do and listen to ways they cope with the weight gain, mood swings or increased appetite that are side effects of the drug is a valuable way to understand why you feel the way you do and maybe even help you find another way to cope with the side effect in a more positive manner. Communicating with another diabetic is a way to learn the following; (1) how someone else in your situation deals with the bruises from the insulin injections. I learned the trick of using an alcohol pad to clean the area before the injection and then using a piece of dry tissue to wipe any blood initiated. Using the alcohol pad after the injection will not allow the blood to clot properly thus easing the possibility of bruising; and (2) how to be able to take your insulin when you eat out.

Understanding what and why you feel like you do is something only someone else who walks in your shoes can provide. When you have the opportunity, take advantage of it.

I want to stress when I say other patients are the best resources in regard to coping with the daily struggles you face, I mean just what I say - coping. Do not use any information from another patient and change your treatments without consulting your doctor. The same is true for any information you obtain over the Internet. Your doctor is the person who knows your history and how you've responded to medications in the past. Only your doctor should dictate your treatments. Feel free to talk to him/her regarding what you learned and if you decide to try something you obtained from another patient, make sure you keep your doctor aware. The objective is to gain as much knowledge and understanding about your health condition or medications so that you can cope with your daily life in a more positive manner and work with your doctor to tweak your treatments based on how you react as an individual. Other patients provide support - your doctor provides treatment.

A word of warning regarding anything you obtain over the Internet. Just as in the real world please do not believe or take as written in stone everything you read on the Internet. People and information on the Internet are from the same source as everything else in this world - people. Anyone can develop a web site and add any information they want. It's an excellent place for scammers as well. It's no different than someone calling yon on the phone or talking to you on the street, do not give anyone your personal information such as social security number, bank accounts, credit card accounts or anything else that could be used in a fraudulent manner to rip you off.

As with all information find out the source and how credible it is. What experience do they have on the subject, are there any alternative motives for using the information, is there money to be made or other advantages gained by your following the information? Unfortunately there are a lot of individuals and groups who will take advantage of desperate people honestly trying to seek information to better their lives. Frustrated patients with diseases like sarcoidosis, cancer or diabetes can be vulnerable to someone promising relief or a cure - for a fee. Common sense and communications with your doctor are the keys to success on the Internet in regard to learning about your conditions or medications. Treat the Internet as you would anything in person and it will be a valuable source of unlimited information.

If you don't have a computer at home don't fear you won't be left out. Visit your local public library, as they will have computers with Internet access available (normally free of charge) along with someone who can guide you as to how to get started. Technology today is nothing like it was even a few years ago when only a geek (for lack of a better term we can all relate to) could maneuver successful on the Internet. Even if you've never used the Internet before in a matter of minutes you can learn the basics to obtain the information you need to better understand your situation. If you can't use a computer based on another health or personal reason, have a loved one or caregiver gather the information for you. Don't allow your fear of technology or inexperience to keep you from information that could improve your quality of life.

Good old fashion books are a resource that could provide benefit to your research as well. Although most new information is put on the Internet, in today's world reading is still a primary and reliable method for obtaining information. Plus, since you're reading this book, it's something you obviously do anyway. A magazine is another resource. It seems there is a magazine for every subject available on the newsstand or in the public library and the articles in current magazines are up to date. Of course, as with seemingly everything, the same magazine is usually available on the Internet as well.

There's another excellent resource I know without a doubt is available to 99% of the American population and that's television. There are a number of cable channels such as the "Learning Channel" or "Discovery Channel" (to name a couple and I'm not promoting either) that have programs relating to health conditions and treatments. The growing number of national/network news stations has programs relating to a variety of health conditions, treatments and issues as well. Your local newscast normally has a health reporter and segment that covers local health news. Maybe you can contact them about your health questions and who knows you might even have your story aired.

Often accompanying the health programs and news stories there will be a more detailed version on the station's Internet web site. In fact a lot of times the guest or source of the story will be available for e-mail questions or live online conversations. This is true with a majority of the magazines with health related stories as well.

Another source you might not think about is your insurance company. When most of us think insurance we think after the fact, and for the most part frustration. We are finally starting to see a trend where the insurance industry is seeing the financial benefits of prevention as opposed to treatment. It's like your car. If you spend a few dollars keeping the oil changed and doing preventive maintenance, you will avoid having to spend the big bucks associated with preventable repairs down the road, so to speak. Your health is no different. Insurance companies today have programs setup to manage conditions such as diabetes, heart problems, and other conditions that can be controlled with proper steps which include diet tips, exercise options, and support groups to help individuals stick to their goals, since it can be extremely hard controlling certain aspects of prevention alone. Use all of the resources available to you because, as far as insurance is concerned, you're paying for the programs anyway with your premiums. Trust me, if customer's health care continues to need more medical attention, which in turn means more monies paid out by your insurance company, then your premiums will only rise in the future. So if your health issues aren't enough to make you take advantage of the educational opportunities available to you by way of your insurance plans then think about the financial impact and not taking advantage of the programs. As the saying goes, "Money talks!" or in this case "Money motivates!"

Last but not least, once you've obtained information the best way to understand your unique situation and put the information to the best use is, like we discussed in the previous chapter, you must understand your own body and mental makeup. This will determine how you use any information you obtain. Remember the keyword "should" and use your judgment and inner voice to determine what works for you and what doesn't. Without saying your doctor should have major input as well. Keep an open mind and never reject any information without first looking at it objectively. You never know from where your best benefit will come but, I guarantee you, if you wear blinders and proceed through life with a closed mind you will live in negativity.

Once you have acquired an understanding of your physical, mental and financial situation for this moment in time, you're now ready to put your knowledge to positive use. This is where Step-2 comes into play.

Step-2…You must honestly accept your reality!

Now comes what is one of the most difficult things most people, if they are honest with themselves, ever have to do…honestly accepting your reality. Once you completed step-1 and have the best understanding of what you "should" expect from your health conditions, you must look in the mirror and honestly accept your fate. This step is why it's so important to understand and listen to your body because now that you know what you "should" expect you now must determine what you "actually" experience. To accomplish this task you must accept what you physically can and can't do at this point in your life.

If there was ever a time when you're forced to turn a traditional negative into a positive, this is it. It's rather easy to determine and accept what you still can do. You simply attempt the tasks and if you can achieve them without causing you any physical, mental or financial damage then continue to do it. Even if you feel minor negative consequences you can determine if those consequences are worth the pleasure or necessity of doing the task. From there you can either continue the task as normal and just expect the consequence, adjust how you do the task to ease the consequence or do the task less often or with assistance to again ease the consequence. This is a decision each individual will have to make based on what his/her body dictates.

The difficult part of this step and the part that takes a mind adjustment is understanding what you can't do any longer as a result of your health condition. This does not and cannot be a negative experience but instead a reality that will make your life more fulfilling. But first you must change your thought process in regard to the word "can't".

Since we were little kids most of us have been told over and over again that we can do anything in life we put our minds to if we work hard enough to achieve our goal. In fact we probably were scolded if we ever said we couldn't do something, be it in school, athletics or social functions. However, even in normal circumstances, although I understand the logic for instilling this mindset into our children's minds (I did the same with my daughter and will do the same with my granddaughter), it's simply not true. There are some of us who no matter how hard we work or how much we try we just don't have what it takes to be a doctor. No matter how hard we work or how much we try we simply don't have the physical abilities to become a professional athlete. No matter how hard we work or how much we practice and dedicate ourselves, some of us don't have the talent to become a professional singer (I'm definitely included in this group!). The little train might have made it up the hill by telling itself, "I think I can, I think I can, I think I can" but the reality is sometimes due to physical, mental and opportunistic situations, we can't.

A chronic health condition that prevents you from doing those things you used to do is a major cause for depression, not only for the patient but the caregiver as well. It doesn't have to be! In fact understanding and accepting the things you can no longer do will, in turn, make your life a more positive experience. First, however, you must learn to accept your new fate honestly and positively.

I understand all too well this is a difficult thing to do, even for a "Professional Patient" like myself. No matter how long you have been dealing with chronic health conditions or how positive an attitude you try to maintain, not being able suddenly or gradually, to do something you have enjoyed doing can cause an extremely negative feeling that will send you in a state of depression. This is normal; however, it's something you cannot allow to stay with you but a very short period of time.

Here is the basis for the swing from negative to positive. Regardless of what you can't do, there are a large number of other things you can do without causing any harm, physically or mentally, to yourself or your loved ones. In fact you might even enjoy the new activities better than the old ones as long as you keep an open mind and don't condemn the activity before you even get started.

Here are some things that have affected my life which I had to take a long look at myself to understand and accept the fact I simply can't do what I used to do, and by doing so make my life a more positive experience. First there was not being able to play basketball anymore. This might not sound serious to some but to me it was! Basketball was one thing I was good at and in turn got respect as a man (however artificial that might be). I grew up with basketball as a center of my life as my father was a basketball coach and playing basketball was a way I was able to survive the street life to which as a young adult I was attracted. It was also the way I bonded with other men since I don't play golf or go to bars. When I finally realized I wasn't physically able to play basketball, during my late prime, it blew my mind. However I understood my reality and started enjoying long walks to replace the physical activity and still watch basketball on a regular basis. In turn I was okay, although I still dream of being back on the court.

Not being able to work a regular 40-hour job was another task I had to give up as a result of my physical health issues. It took me a long time to accept this fate because I needed to feel in control of myself, to be a provider and make a living. Around the year 2000 my doctors started suggesting I consider filing for disability and stop working full-time. I was missing a lot of work and was having to go out on disability leaves on a regular basis. Family members started mentioning this reality to me as well, but I was having no part of it. I even went back to work early one disability leave against doctor's orders.

Finally in 2002 I was part of a "workforce reduction", which both my employer (who had been extremely supportive since my conditions started in 1986) and I understood was the best move for me. It was a shock at first but over time I've been able to fill my time productively. By honestly accepting the fact I "can't" I'm now able to maintain a positive frame of mind, and better health.

There are so many things in life to do that you should be able to do something productive to help you maintain a positive quality of life from both a physical and mental perspective. On the other hand if you don't honestly accept the fact you can't do something anymore and continue to attempt to do the task, you will only have negative results. You will be frustrated with your inability to perform the task anymore, which will cause a mental breakdown and physical concerns. Depending on the task (take working for example) your inability to perform will cause others depending on you to suffer negatively as well. Anyway you look at it denying your reality only has negative affects. Acknowledging that you can't do something anymore and replacing that task with another or adjusting our lifestyle might be hard at first; however, in the end not only you but your associates, friends and loved ones will benefit in a positive manner as well.

Negatives can be positives when you look at the individual situation without blinders and with an open mind. Keep telling our children they can do anything they put their minds to if they work hard to achieve their goals because it instills a work ethic our young folks need to survive. However, as a patient with a chronic health condition, a caregiver supporting a loved one, or the average adult growing older by the day, you must forget the "I can" mentality and understand, accept and adjust to make "I can't" work in a positive manner for your quality of life.

Step-3…Deal with your current reality!

Once you have an understanding of your health condition and how it or your medications "should" affect you and have honestly accepted what you now can and can't do, then you must live your life to the fullest. The method by which you deal with your unique individual circumstances varies from situation to situation and I'm not even going to attempt to try and give you examples of what you need to do. I will, however, say if you have learned the things it takes to be a successful patient and have completed steps 1 and 2, you will know for yourself what you need to do.

Your objective is simple - do what it takes to live a long, healthy, and fulfilling life. Your health is the most important thing in your earthly life, before family, your profession, personal activities or financial issues. Without your health you have nothing. It's your responsibility to ensure you do whatever it takes to live your life as healthy as possible. It will be difficult at times and achieving anything I've discussed thus far will take dedication, frustration, and will power but the results for yourself, your family, your professional life, and the possible financial benefits are worth every effort.

Like most things in life there's always a wrench thrown into the equation, so look out because here it comes. Once you have achieved steps 1, 2, and 3 parts of your life will change and you will be back at the beginning. Change is a fact of life and a source of frustration until we learn to deal with it in a positive manner. It's also something most people have problems with. Changes in processes, procedures or even how the new print on your local Sunday newspaper looks are things to which you have to adjust. Some people initially fight the change or are overwhelmed, until frustration becomes too much. They then realize they have no choice but to adjust or quit. Regardless of their choice at the end of the day the changes are still present, until they change again. All things come to an end at some point in life and something new begins. That's just life!

Your health life is no different, only with health changes you are compelled to adjust immediately, as the results of not adjusting could be life altering, or worse. In other words you have only one logical choice, because not changing is something that cannot be considered. As a result of this fact of life the reality is you must continue to stay on top of your situation, look in the mirror, be honest with yourself and accept your current way of life then deal with it to the best of your ability over and over again.

As everyone else I've had to make many changes in my life, especially since 1986 when my health started to become part of my daily routine. Learning how to adjust to each different change, both the major and seemingly harmless, is something you must determine based on the individual and the specific circumstances. I can't tell you the best way for you to adapt to your changes in life; only you can determine the best course of action for yourself. I can tell you how you adapt to your ever changing reality is one of the most important things you will ever do in life. So please don't ignore change but embrace it. You have no other logical choice!

One of the hardest things I've had to adjust to recently is taking insulin. As I mentioned earlier I'm scared to death of needles so giving myself daily injections scared the hell out of me. My blood sugar levels started maintaining a level that was over the range sugar levels should exceed (170 and up) on a regular basis. My endocrinologist knew of my fear so he tried to work with me by trying other options. We tried taking a couple of oral medications before my meals. One caused me to swell up, much like the prednisone, especially in my eyes. It got to the point my eyes were almost swollen shut.

The other didn't have much of a positive effect either as my sugar levels started to stay in the low to mid 200 ranges on a regular basis. Even first thing in the morning when blood sugar levels are the lowest due to fasting over night, my sugar levels averaged between 175 and 200 every morning. I would make any excuse I could not to have to take insulin. I would tell my endocrinologist I didn't want to try anything new when I was out of town (I was spending a lot of time in Florida with my father at this time in my life) and I would walk more and watch my diet. I wouldn't even check my blood sugar levels or certainly not check them three or four times a day as I was instructed. Then I would say I forgot to bring the results with me when I was suppose to provide them to him. I know…BAD PATIENT and it went against everything I knew was my responsibility!

The reality was the only person I was hurting was myself. I understood what diabetes could cause me in my life and that scared me as well. The last thing I want is to go blind or lose the ability to walk, but neither scared me at the time more than injecting myself. Even when I found out the option for taking the insulin was a pen, as opposed to a syringe, I still couldn't honestly accept my new reality. Finally, after my blood sugar levels started averaging in the mid to high 200 range my endocrinologist put his foot down. He asked me the age old question, "What is your goal in life?" Without giving me an opportunity to answer he said, "To live as long as you can and as healthy as you can. You won't accomplish either if you don't start taking insulin." At this point I knew it was time to accept this change in my life and do what I had to do.

I started by taking a few units of Levemir insulin at 8:30 in the evening, which I administered by using a flex pen, and I was still taking an oral medication before each meal. This insulin would provide me with a steady flow of insulin for 24 hours. The nurse showed me how to administer the injection and gave me another valuable tip, which was to use the mini-needles, as they would cause me less pain and bruising. After a couple of weeks and no real improvement, as my A1C levels or blood sugar levels remained well above the normal range of 7 A1C % or 170mg/dl for blood sugar readings, in fact I was averaging higher than 9 A1C% or 240mg/dl blood sugar reading, my endocrinologist raised the dosage. It was time for me to do what I had to do before it was too late. Finally, I honestly accepted my reality.

I started taking an injection of 30 units of Levemir in the morning and evening. I also stopped taking the oral medication before my meals and started taking an injection of NovoLog insulin, the insulin that works immediately for an hour or so, before each meal and evening snack. The number of units was determined by what my blood sugar level was before each meal. Needless to say this has been an ongoing adjustment from a physical, mental, and medication aspect – a complete lifestyle adjustment.

Now I must remember to have my insulin with me when I'm out as well as taking my blood sugar levels before each meal and snack. Of course I still watch what and when I eat along with walking regularly, even on those days I don't really feel like it. I must also learn to deal with feeling like a pen cushion in my thighs and stomach. When you take five to six injections (I know to some that might not sound like a lot but for someone scared of needles, well it's a lot!) you run out of places to inject yourself that aren't already sore. My reality now dictates this is what I must do and as hard as it was initially it proves we as human beings can adapt to anything when we have to. Life goes on. You either live it or, we don't want to even think of the "or".

Learning to be a successful patient takes a lot of effort on the patient's part and is a continuous, ever changing experience. Once you have learned what it takes to be a patient along with learning the 3-step philosophy, you now have a good foundation for success regardless of your health conditions, be it temporary, chronic or life-threatening. You now have a good foundation for success as a patient; however, there's so much more to deal with in today's medical environment in order to be successful and get the benefits for which you're entitled.

...4...

Learn all you can about your current health situation, honestly accept your reality and then deal with it by any means necessary to ensure you live a positive quality of life for yourself and your family. Without your health you have nothing!

5
What A Difference A Doctor Makes!

Although there are a lot of factors in today's medical environment to ensure success, along with a multitude of things an individual must learn and adjust to from a patient's perspective, one thing still remains the same throughout medical history - your doctor is the most important resource a patient has in regard to treating and maintaining one's health. The patient/doctor relationship is still, and always will be, at the forefront of the prevention, diagnosis, treatment, and healing processes. The success of the relationship will have a tremendous impact on a patient's quality of life. As with everything regarding an individual's health life, it's the patient's responsibility to ensure this vital relationship is a positive marriage.

When you stop and think about it the patient/doctor relationship is basically, in theory, a marriage of sorts. I once had a conversation with my endocrinologist in 2005 regarding my father being admitted into hospice care as a result of his battle with cancer. He made a statement to me that made a lot of sense in regard to the patient/doctor relationship. He told me, "Having to put someone in hospice can actually be harder on the family than on the patients themselves. In fact, it can be extremely hard on us doctors as well. When you treat someone for a long period of time, say as I've treated you, we become like family. I just put someone in hospice I've been treating for over 20 years and it affected me tremendously emotionally, as if they were part of my immediate family. After all, doctors are human too!"

In a lot of cases your doctor is going to know almost as much about your most personal details than your spouse. In fact they may even know some things your spouse doesn't know, healthwise that is. They're going to see you on good days and your worst. All of the aspects of any relationship are present with great personal consequences riding on every result. Treat the relationship with the importance it mandates.

Developing a successful patient/doctor relationship doesn't happen overnight and like even the best of marriages will take time and constant work to be truly successful. The first step is choosing the right doctor for your needs. Where do you begin?

There are several factors individuals will look at when choosing a doctor. Some look at location and convenience. Is the doctor close to their home or place of employment? Is he/she available for appointments after normal business hours or early morning? What emergency facility are they associated with and how close is that facility, or a branch, to your home, possible a big deal with today's insurance requirements? These are some questions that might determine the doctor you choose.

Some folks look at the personal traits of a doctor when deciding whom to try. What is his/her sex, age, religion, race or nationality? Personally I don't use personal traits as a factor. My endocrinologist is an Arab-American male about 12 years older than me, my current PCP is an African-American male, probably around my own age or a few years older, and my dentist is a Caucasian male about my age or a few years younger. The best PCP with whom I was most comfortable with and had a tremendous amount of success at a time when I was experiencing a multitude of problems was a Caucasian female, a few years younger than myself. The only reason I had to switch doctors was the fact she left her practice to run a Detroit inner city health clinic providing health care to those without insurance coverage. My specialists and pharmacists have been of a diverse age, race and sex. Even though I've had problems over the years with every personal trait, I have found these traits have no input on the quality of care I received or on how I am able to interact in regard to my own health treatments. I believe everyone is equal and the traits of the individual determine his/her ability to obtain success from a doctor's service.

On the other hand I can understand how some might feel more comfortable with someone who might have personal traits as themselves. For example a female patient might feel more comfortable undressing in front of a female doctor or discussing sensitive problems as opposed to a male. A male might feel more comfortable talking about male hormone issues with another male. A patient from the inner city might feel more comfortable with a doctor with the same background or you could reverse it and say a patient from a small town might not feel comfortable with someone from the big city. You might feel an older doctor has more experience, although they might be set in their own ways while a younger doctor is more open minded and has the benefit of training with modern technology however actual experience, a vital advantage, is lacking. The important thing is a patient, like a spouse with their mate, must be comfortable with their doctor in order to build a successful relationship and in turn get successful results. I would advise you not to be too hung up on personal traits, as the objective of this relationship is strictly business, the business of maintaining your quality of life as a result of maintaining your health. Never lose site of the objective!

My primary goal for choosing a doctor is the qualifications they have and my medical needs. Getting referrals from others who have used them is a good source for choosing a doctor. A word of warning I've learned the hard way…be careful when using referrals unless you learn to ask the right questions first. Just because someone else has success with a doctor doesn't mean you will. Personalities, that of the patient who is referring the doctor, the actual doctor, and your own comes into play when determining compatibility. Like physical personal traits and how we feel from a comfort level is unique, so are personalities and how we as individuals interact with each other. This is something you will address and in turn grow together as a team once you've started building your relationship with your new doctor. First impressions tell a lot but successful relationships are built with time.

The main factor you want to compare when considering a referral is what I've previously described - how did the patient giving you the referral actually use the doctor services? This is one reason why I take some of the responsibility for my failed experiences and results associated with the seven doctors and five years it took to diagnose my sarcoidosis while I continued to get sicker by the day. I didn't know to ask the important questions when given referrals associates.

The perfect example was the seventh doctor, the one with the "move back to Florida solution". At the time I was desperate and at the end of my rope. My manager referred me to this doctor with confidence on his part. He told me how easy he was to talk to, how thorough he was, what positive results this doctor had diagnosed for him as he went on and on with positive talk. I should have known better to ask him anyway because my manager was one of those self-centered individuals.

Always understand the source of your information! After my disastrous appointment I asked my manager in more detail what specifically had the doctor done for him? I learned my manager had only seen him one time for a physical for which nothing was found and no follow-up instructions were given. This was the extent of my manager's relationship with this doctor. See the importance of understanding your source and asking the right questions beforehand? Yeah I take some responsibility for my lack of knowledge but one thing's for sure - I suffered all of the results!

There are resources for referrals other than patients. I'm sure you have seen them advertised on television or in paper media. Some that comes to mind are 1-800-DENTIST for dentist or even 1-800-LAW-YERS for attorneys (I'm not endorsing either of these services nor have I used either. They just happen to be a couple currently with a lot of television commercials in the Detroit area.). These services usually do a screening process on their members, although the same questions still need to be asked since each patient's situation is unique. You can request a doctor based on location, specialty, insurance acceptance, male or female, hours of operation or other factors as well. It's a good way to get referrals if you don't know anyone to ask or want to keep your health needs private.

One thing to keep in mind with these services is they only refer you to their members and it usually costs the doctor something in order to join. A good example for me is my dentist. I had a specific referral that would save me money (I don't remember the details as it was around 1992) but when I called to see if they participated, they didn't because it ended up costing them too much money and a restriction of patients. My point is although they have a wide range of doctors to refer they still might not have the right one for you. Legwork on your part is still the best option.

Your insurance company is another resource you can use for choosing a doctor. With this option keep in mind it's business with the insurance company, therefore, they're going to refer doctors who participate in their plans and play by their rules. Most insurance plans offer a variety of good doctors, although you usually have to pick a certain facility with which they are associated or else pay a higher out of pocket cost (Tier Pricing, as it's normally called). Regardless of your referral from other patients at the end of the day, you must highly consider your insurance coverage and financial situation options.

Outside of the fact your insurance company might limit your choices, reality might dictate limited choices as well. If you live in a rural area, your choices are going to be more limited than those in an urban area. Choice is one area in which the patient/doctor relationship differs from a spouse. If the choices for a spouse are limited, you just stay single, which might be a little lonely but won't alter your quality of life or possibly kill you. However, with a doctor, lack of choice and doing without is not an option. We all must deal with a doctor more than once in our lifetime. Ignoring our health problems will, without a doubt, alter our quality of life and speed up our lifespan on earth. The important thing is when you do decide or must choose a specific doctor enter the relationship with an open mind and willingness to build a positive relationship. It's always your, and only yours, health at stake.

Once you've made your decision regarding which doctor you want to use it's time to start building a successful relationship. Building and maintaining a successful relationship with anyone in your life takes a lot of effort and work from all parties, even if the personalities are compatible. As with any relationship, marriage, friendship, business or medical, the most important aspect is honest communication from all parties. It's important to remember when building any relationship that relationships are a two way street and honest communication is more than just speaking your mind or your point of view. Honest communication takes listening with an open mind, expressing directly what's on your mind and what you're feeling, without the pressure of feeling guilty or embarrassed, and knowing what you're expressing is being taken seriously, without prejudice. As simple as it may sound, honest communication is probably one of the hardest things to do in life, especially when it comes to your health.

Regardless of how intelligent or experienced your doctor may be, he/she will never be able to read a patient's mind and know how to treat him/her unless the patient honestly communicates what the patient is specifically feeling. It simply can't be done! A patient must be comfortable enough with his/her doctor to tell the whole truth and nothing but the truth without holding anything back or crying wolf. Every detail is important and could have an impact on how you're successfully treated. You simply cannot allow fear of the unknown or being afraid of what it might take to cure you to keep you from honestly telling your doctor what's going on with you healthwise. You must never allow a possible need for sympathy or attention to allow you to exaggerate what symptoms you're experiencing or how bad those symptoms are affecting your health. I'll say it again, the truth, the whole truth, and nothing but the truth is the only option you have if you want successful results.

The second part of the communication process is for your doctor to listen to what you're saying without prejudice or thinking he/she already knows what you're going to say. It doesn't matter if he/she has heard it a million times each patient is unique and if the doctor doesn't listen with his/her total attention then the one unique symptom this individual patient is experiencing that could alter the treatment might be missed. There is no place for ego on either side in a patient/doctor relationship!

Once you've told the doctor your symptoms and the doctor has listened attentively the process reverses itself. Now it's the doctor's time to talk and time for the patient to listen. This is the basis for all honest communications and in the patient/doctor relationship it will dramatically affect the results of the treatment. A doctor can only look for diseases and treat symptoms described to him/her by the patient, and the patient can only get better if he/she listens to the doctor's instructions. Honest communication is the start, ongoing and end to building a positive patient/doctor relationship.

Another trait that is built from honest communications and is a requirement in order to achieve success is trust. Without trust you can't have honest communications; without honest communications you can't have trust, and without both you can't have a successful patient/doctor relationship. Having trust in your doctor and your doctor having trust in his/her patient is mandatory for success! After all, your doctor is going to give you advice that, in turn, you must follow, which will have an immediate and long-term effect on your life. That advice is going to come based on what you tell your doctor. Without trust you will not feel comfortable enough to tell your doctor all that's wrong with you and that mistake could have dramatic affects on your quality of life. Having the trust in your doctor, and those others in your life, to tell the whole truth about what you feel is a vital step in getting the support and care you need.

As the patient you must not only be honest and upfront about your health but about other things in your life as well. I can't stress enough the importance all aspects of your life has on your overall health. You must develop a relationship with your doctor, another prime use of the term marriage, to discuss certain personal aspects of your life that might not directly relate to your health but, without a doubt, indirectly relate to the success of your treatment.

Here are some examples of situations in your life, outside your direct health symptoms, that have an impact on your health. One major impact is financial issues. If you're under financial stress or hardships it affects your mental state. Fear of losing your job or of becoming victim of a corporate downsizing and not knowing where your next mortgage payment is coming from has a direct impact on your health. If you're going through home foreclosure as so many Americans of all walks of life are doing today then other health issues might arise from the stress you're experiencing. Although you might not see your financial state as the doctor's business, in reality it is. You don't have to go into detail and obviously aren't looking to your doctor for financial advice but you must make them aware of your state of mind and the pressure you're under as a result of financial problems. People tend to underestimate the power and the role these issues play in their overall life.

Other life situations that have an impact of your health are family relationship problems such as going through a divorce or having issues raising children. Having a death in the family or having a loved one fall seriously ill can alter your health as well and should be mentioned to your doctor. Maybe you've taking college classes where the grades will determine a financial or career result. Are you unhappy in your current employment, living environment or feeling you're being pulled from all ends by family, work, and financial responsibilities? Bottom line is you must develop trust through honest communications in order to feel comfortable informing your doctor of these life situations and let your doctor determine the impact they have on your treatments.

Stress has a powerful impact on your overall health! My endocrinologist told me something with which I strongly agree; stress isn't the health problem but stress brings out other health problems that already exist. How those health problems are treated could depend on the stress causing them. It could be as simple as changing a life style or doing something to relieve the stress level, if possible. On the other hand, the stress might mean the patient needs to treat the health problem more aggressively while his/her life situation straightens itself out. Bottom line is without the honest communications and trust between patient and doctor, a wild goose chase might develop with you the patient feeling the negative consequences. Be honest and don't put yourself in that situation!

You must be able to talk openly with your doctor about things that have an impact on your physical and mental health. Financial issues and the impact of health care are one of the issues you must not be embarrassed to discuss. I have already told you about the story of the chiropractor that without our honest communications regarding costs, would have never successfully treated my migraines.

We all must understand doctors, like anyone else who works, work for money. After all it is a profession. However, a good doctor will not be unreasonable and will be flexible in regard to money issues affecting a treatment, if you're upfront with them about your financial situation. Here's another example of success directly related to my positive long-term relationship with my endocrinologist. My insurance company dictates that my bi-weekly depo-testosterone injection be given by my PCP in order to cover it. After my long-time PCP left for her new opportunity and I was searching for a replacement, I began to have a lot of billing errors and hassles in regard to getting my injection. I had almost reached the point I was ready to leave the network, even if it meant leaving my endocrinologist. I told him of my frustrations, and he simply smiled and told me to start coming to his office and he would give me the injection for free without billing my insurance. He wasn't worried about the $6 an injection the insurance company paid him ($156 per year) or of the minor expense of using 26 syringes a year. His concern was to relieve my frustration.

If a doctor won't listen to your financial needs or make any adjustments to work with you in order to better serve your health care needs, then you've probably picked the wrong doctor. Keep in mind it's still business and sometimes the doctor's hands might be tied, but if he/she won't listen to you and attempt to meet you half way, then how are you going to have the trust in him/her to discuss other situations that might have a major impact on your health?

Therefore, as a patient it's mandatory you have a comfort level, built on honest communications and the trust in knowing your doctor listens to your best interest and unique situation are all that matters. Without the two-way honesty and mutual trust between patient and doctor how could any success be obtained? All aspects of our life affect our health. There is no manual or carved in stone procedure or process on how to treat an individual patient. The patient must provide the input, the doctor the output and together the positive results are fine-tuned. Without honest communications and trust, the basics of any successful relationship, this positive success cannot be obtained.

From honest communications and trust comes respect. Respect is critical in the ultimate patient/doctor relationship. Sometimes we hit it off with individuals from the start and sometimes it takes a while to warm up to some people while some of us never connect. The patient/doctor relationship is no different. We're both human beings. Remember when choosing and building a relationship with your doctor it is always business and not personal. At the same time, however, you must have some personal connection in order for honest communications and trust to develop into respect. This is why the "bedside manner", so it's called, of a doctor is important.

Speaking of bedside manner, I would like to recommend a movie I think all patients, and even more so, doctors should watch. To take it a step farther I think all interns should be required not only to watch this movie as a part of their training but also to go through some of the situations a patient must experience in order to truly understand how their actions affect other people, from both a health and mental perspective. The doctor should understand the discomfort of some of those procedures he/she finds necessary to put a patient through, thus giving a better ability to better relieve the anxiety of the patient, thereby, promoting more positive results.

The movie, available on DVD, is entitled, "The Doctor" and stars William Hurt as a doctor who thought he knew it all. In time the shoe is on the other foot, as he became the patient with a life threatening disease. His perspective on life and the medical environment became quite different then! There's one scene where he's given the wrong (uncomfortable) test and, in the context of the movie, you find yourself glad. However, the reality is it happens in real life more than we want to admit, and in the reality context there's nothing funny about it, even to an arrogant know-it-all. Check it out. I think you'll find it of interest.

Choosing the correct doctor is one of the most important choices you'll make in life. Building a positive relationship with him/her will be even harder, as all relationships are. You don't have to like your doctor as a friend or want to hang out with him/her, but you do have to feel comfortable enough with his/her personally to open up and trust him/her enough to follow the treatments they provide. Your inner voice will supply you with direction so listen to your instincts.

The impact of your choice of doctors is dramatic in regard to the quality of life for not only you, but your family as well. Even if you aren't suffering from any known illnesses today, remember it only takes a second for your life to change from a health standpoint. So regardless, if you're healthy or suffering from a chronic health condition take choosing and building a successful relationship with your doctor seriously.

Also, like all relationships, sometimes it just doesn't work out. Patient/doctor relationships are no different. There can be a multitude of reasons for the misconnection - you might not feel comfortable personally with your doctor for various reasons; you might feel your doctor doesn't listen to you or rushes you in and out of your appointments; you might not be satisfied with the follow-up or lack of follow-up you receive; you might have problems with the doctor's staff or billing practices; you might feel your doctor won't ask for help when needed; or you simply aren't getting positive results. These are just a few of the reasons that could cause a patient/doctor relationship to go sour. Whether it's an abusive marriage or a patient/doctor relationship going through the motions with no success, don't be afraid to leave and start over.

I understand it's frustrating to build positive relationships and starting over is a scary thing to think about. To add to the urgency with patient/doctor relationships, as opposed to a marriage after divorce, you can't take your time to find a new doctor as you can to find a new spouse. Your search must start immediately. Don't let the fear of the unknown or hearing what you want to hear keep you in a relationship that only causes you more health problems. Everyone likes to hear good results but when those good results are wrong it only increases the chances your health will suffer unjustly in the future, maybe for your lifetime. Not having the confidence, knowledge and energy, and also fearing what you don't want to hear can keep you hoping what you are being told is true even though your body tells you it is not. Look at my pre-sarcoidosis diagnosis period from 1986 till 1991. Don't allow my experience to become yours!

There are a ton of good and excellent doctors of all sexes, races, nationalities, ages, backgrounds, religions, specialties, locations, insurance programs, and personalities available in today's medical environment. It's up to you to find the one for you and start building a positive relationship. One thing is for sure; the consequences will always fall back on the patient. As you would choose your soul mate carefully, do everything in your power to build a successful marriage while facing an ever changing reality on a daily basis, do the same with your doctor relationship as well. You have too much at stake not to!

...5...

The basis for any successful relationship, patient/doctor relationships included, is honest communications between all parties and trust, which in turn develops respect. Choosing the correct doctor is a decision not to be taken lightly. Building a positive relationship takes continuous work from all parties in order to be successful. For the patient the result of the relationship's success fall entirely on his/her shoulders!

6
The Appointment

One of the most important aspects for being a successful patient is learning how to take advantage of your one on one opportunity with your doctor. This is the time in which you must communicate, trust, understand, and benefit from your doctor. It's extremely important you make the most of the opportunity - the first time!

To start, you must remember and implement into your visit an important requirement for learning how to be a successful patient - be prepared to wait. Over time you will get better at waiting. Depending on how you feel will determine how patient you're able to wait. I can't emphasize how important learning to be patient while waiting to be called in to see the doctor, with more waiting once again in the examining room, is to the success of your visit. You can't be full of attitude or frustrated to the point you just want to leave once you have the opportunity to discuss your health in person with your doctor. In order to have successful results and maintain a positive relationship you can't allow negative emotions to take over your common sense.

My philosophy is I don't mind waiting as long as when I see the doctor I get his/her uninterrupted attention for as long as it's needed to cover my health issues. If not, then I have a problem not only with the wait but also the ability of the doctor to properly treat whatever is troubling me at the time. That's the proper time to complain and take action to correct the problem.

Another thing to remember while waiting is that when you're with the doctor one on one the objective of the appointment is to discuss your health situation, diagnose any problems, and then come up with a treatment plan. It is not a social visit! Don't think because you had to wait a while and you now have the doctor's full attention this is the time for a variety of small talk. Get to the business of your health. There was a reason why you waited so long. There are other patients waiting as you did, and the doctor's time is valuable, as is yours and the waiting patients.

I understand some folks like to feel friendly with their doctor. This was high on my father's list and usually the first thing he would comment on regarding a new doctor. It's also a valuable skill for a doctor to have good bedside manner and to make their patient feel comfortable with him/her by adding the personal touch while still taking care of the business at hand. It makes sense too. You, as a human being, will be more likely to be honest about your issues, both healthwise and personal, with someone you feel friendly. A good technique as long as everyone remembers the objective of the appointment is business, not social.

There is a difference in spending time discussing financial, relationship or employment matters in your life, as they can have an impact on your health, than spending time talking in detail about how your favorite sports team is doing this season or what movies you've seen as those subjects have no impact on your health situation at all. Again I understand being friendly matters to some and this is strictly my personality speaking out. Sometimes it takes those types of conversations to open up the more relevant health related exchanges of information. It is also important for a doctor to understand each patient's individual makeup to get the most success out of the relationship. For some, a little unrelated small talk might be positive and for others like myself, not necessary. What is important is getting the benefits of your health situation in a short period of time. To accomplish this success preparation is the key.

One of the best tools for making sure you're prepared and not forget to tell the doctor anything going on regarding your health is to write down all of your symptoms and concerns, and then provide them at the beginning of the appointment. I can't begin to tell you the number of times doctors have thanked me for providing them a written list so they can see in black and white what's going on with their patient. The list can be typed or a handwritten note, a full sheet of paper or a small notebook pad sheet, the original or a photocopy - just make sure you provide a list.

To compile the list you should always keep notes anytime something affects your health between appointments. Write down everything immediately because if you don't, you will probably forget or forget certain details, especially if you start feeling better. Just because you might feel better temporarily doesn't mean the problem has gone away. When it's time for your appointment put everything into a list. Don't leave certain things out because you think they aren't important. If it affected your health it could be important. That's why you're seeing the doctor, remember?

Also, please do not let fear have an impact on what you put on your list. I don't know why we, and we all do it, including myself, think a symptom will go away on its own without getting worse or causing other preventable health problems. If the symptom has gotten to the point you feel pain, then it's a problem that needs to be mentioned. It's human nature to be afraid and avoid possible negative results. That's why some people wait to even go to the doctor, and especially the dentist, until the pain is unbearable. Just as the insurance companies wake up to the fact prevention saves money, you too, must understand telling your doctor about all issues upfront will avoid preventable pain, as well as prevent loss of out-of-pocket money, and ensure a better quality of life while minimizing health related hardships in your future. It's not your call as to what's important but it is your responsibility to yourself, your family, and your doctor to be honest about any and everything regarding your health.

I can give you a couple of personal examples for myself regarding outside issues affecting my overall health. First, when I was dealing with my mother-in-law and my father both battling cancer, my emotions were running wild and I felt pulled from all sides. I remember one night taking my wife to the emergency room and staying all night, getting home the next morning, I had to keep my commitment to my mother-in-law to take her to her appointment that morning so we could talk to her doctors regarding her radiation and chemotherapy treatments. I dropped my wife at our house and immediately went to pick up my mother-in-law. My health suffered a few days from that experience but it was something I had to do. I remember taking my father everyday for six weeks to Tallahassee for radiation treatments (a three plus hour overall process). Some mornings I would feel terrible not only because of the stress of the unknown, but also knowing when I got back to Perry there were other issues I needed to address, as well as with missing my wife back in Detroit. These additional situations in my life were causing me to struggle healthwise. Stress brings out what's already wrong with you so my endocrinologist made a few temporary adjustments, like slightly increasing my prednisone, to help me cope with my current personal situations.

Another example was a tooth that was giving me a lot of trouble. In fact I eventually had it removed. During the time of the irritation, like most individuals, I put off the dental trip as long as I could, but I started experiencing other health related problems. I told my endocrinologist about the tooth and he decided before he changed my medications we would wait and see how I felt after the tooth was extracted. As soon as the tooth was gone my other heath problems went away as well. Even though my dental problems weren't the responsibility of my endocrinologist, by making him aware of it he was able to better understand the health problems for which he was responsible. I'll discuss the importance of your dental health later on.

One of the problems with fear in regard to disclosing everything bothering your health to your doctor is you have a tendency to hear what you want to hear. We've all done it. You tell the doctor something that's wrong, and the doctor doesn't think it's too serious or tells you to keep doing what you're doing and on the next appointment we'll see how it's going. You're so relieved with the fact you don't have to increase medications or do any tests (I did this over and over to avoid insulin) that you, either consciously or subconsciously, leave the appointment without mentioning other issues you have. When you provide a list at the beginning of the appointment, it not only eliminates this from happening but could have an impact on the initial issue as well. Either way your doctor has your complete information to consider which, in turn, gives him/her the knowledge to prescribe a more successful treatment.

Aside from the health issues be sure, as we previously discussed, to mention any outside situations in your life that could impact how your body is reacting at this time. Remember to keep it to the point, as the objective is to let your doctor know of other impact issues not start a social conversation. If your doctor needs more detail he/she will ask.

Something else of extreme importance to include on your list is how you have reacted to any previously prescribed medications or treatments and if you have actually done as the doctor suggested. It's dangerous to your health to not be completely honest about this subject, even if you get a stern lecture in return. Your doctor has to work with the correct information or else he/she will prescribe another medication or treatment based on false information, and that's not good.

Let me ask you a question. Let's say your doctor tells you to take 20MGs of a specific medication once a day. You take the medication for a couple of days then quit. When you have your next appointment the following month and you're asked how did the medication work, instead of being honest and saying you only took it a couple of days, you just say you feel the same. As a result of your information the doctor now prescribes 40MGs of a stronger medication to be taken twice a day. You leave the appointment and take the medication the next day as instructed and have a critical reaction because the medication was too strong for your condition. Who's at fault? Your doctor, who prescribed the medication based on your information that the other medication had no effect, or you, who didn't tell the doctor the truth? We know who felt the consequences!

Control is an unwritten factor that's associated with a doctor's appointment as well and must be overcome in order to have honest communications and positive results. I think this is one reason why a few, not all, doctors have ego issues and why a few, not all, patients feel intimidated by their doctors to the point they don't tell everything that's wrong with them.

On the surface it looks as if the doctor is in complete control of the patient once the examining room door is closed. It's the doctor who asks the majority of the questions and gives the instructions as to what happens in the appointment. The doctor will have you take off your clothes and get into some very awkward positions then perform some painful tests. Your doctor will see you in positions your own spouse has never seen. Now that's control, or is it?

The reality is the patient is actually the one in control. This is something you must never lose sight of. First of all your doctor cannot force you to do anything against your will. If you're uncomfortable with a test being performed ask for an explanation as to why this test is needed. If you're still uncomfortable ask for a second opinion. No doctor should ever get an attitude or have any reservation in regard to a patient asking for a second opinion about anything regarding his/her medical treatment. If the doctor does - leave immediately!

If you're uncomfortable being alone with the doctor, especially if you're undressed and the doctor is of a different sex, ask for someone of your sex to be in the room while the exam is being conducted. If all information verifies an uncomfortable tests needs to be performed tell yourself that you're allowing this to be done to you. You are in control of your health situation at all times.

Once again trust is a major factor in regard to a patient/doctor relationship and the success of any appointment. Trust is what allows a patient to put themselves in uncomfortable positions, as they trust in their doctor's ability to treat them successfully based on the results of the uncomfortable test. The reality is a lot of necessary medical tests are painful and uncomfortable to the patient. Even an understanding, gentle doctor with whom you have complete trust in can't avoid the discomfort and painful aspects of certain required tests. They simply have to be performed. Just keep telling yourself, even if you're scared or nervous, you're allowing this test to be performed on you. You are in control!

Embarrassment is another emotion that needs to be left in the waiting room. There is nothing embarrassing about a medical condition or symptom. It's a medical condition! Communicate with trust your medical problem to the doctor so you can get treatment that will get you back to normal. Not telling your doctor doesn't make the problem go away but only increases the chance it will get serious and other health problems will follow.

Sexual problems, especially for males, are health problems most men will keep to themselves. There's nothing embarrassing about any health problem, sexual problems included. Let's say you have a problem where you can't perform sexually anymore. Would you rather keep the problem to yourself and avoid sexual pleasure or tell your doctor, and get a simple treatment that allows you to make love again with your lover? Do you realize how many men and women have sexual issues that can easily be corrected if they would just tell their doctors the truth? If you can't honestly communicate with your doctor and trust that they will make the right decision, or ask for help if they don't know exactly what to do, then you're with the wrong doctor.

Here's another advantage in regard to providing your doctor with the written list before an appointment starts that could help you determine how effective the communication is between the two of you. If you have five issues on your list and after reading the list at the start of the appointment your doctor only addresses three, you have a problem! Your doctor isn't listening to you and therefore can't properly treat your health situation - end of story!

I had a perfect example of this with a doctor around 1999. I was looking for a replacement PCP to replace my longtime PCP who left her practice to run a Detroit medical clinic. My endocrinologist had referred this doctor to me. My first appointment was more like a business meeting to determine if he thought he could handle my health situation. I always have my endocrinologist refer my PCP because I need a PCP for insurance requirements, but my endocrinologist is in reality my primary doctor. That's why I use one he works with, or usually was an intern under him at some point during his/her residency, so they won't have any problems referring me to him for constant treatment and the communication process between them is good.

On my second appointment I provided the doctor with a list of four issues with which I was having problems. He looked at the note and complimented me on providing my issues upfront. He put the note down and proceeded to hurry through the first two issues. He then got up and was heading for the door concluding our appointment. I stopped him by asking what about the other two issues? He checked my folder for the note and said, "Oh yeah." He asked me a couple of seemingly unrelated questions and told me I was okay. He never even moved a step away from the door as my folder was in his hand. I told the medical assistant there was no need to make a follow-up appointment. I immediately called my endocrinologist for another referral and never returned to that doctor again.

Providing a written note of your symptoms is only the first step. You should also write down the instructions your doctor gives for treatment. You might think you understand and will remember at the time of the appointment, and you're probably ready to get out of there as fast as you can, but for your own sake you need to take the time to ensure you have everything written down. Not to stereotype but...if you don't understand your doctor's handwriting don't hesitate to ask another staff member to rewrite it for you or take your time and write it in your own handwriting. We don't all have good penmanship, nothing to be ashamed of, but it's mandatory you're able to read your notes or else they're useless. Make sure you not only understand what was discussed in your appointment but make sure you have readable notes as well.

As you can see I'm big on writing down anything you want to remember, especially anything affecting your health. When I was in the corporate world I would always take the time to rewrite my notes after a meeting. During the meeting I would write keywords or half sentences that made perfect sense to me at the time. However a month later I wouldn't have a clue what the meaning of the keyword was or what the half sentence was intended to mean. But if I took the time to rewrite the notes in full sentences I understood; then I, or anyone else, could pick up my notes years later and have a perfect understanding of what took place in that particular meeting.

Having detailed notes might take a little extra effort on your part but the benefits down the road are worth every minute you spend. Forgetting one small detail could cause you serious consequences. It will also help when you go to other doctors to have a written account of what you have been instructed by your primary doctor. In fact, when I go to any new doctor or specialist for the first time I take a sheet with all of my health conditions and current medications to accompany my notes of issues to be addressed. Personally I want my doctor to have all of the information possible regarding my health situation in order for him/her to make the best decision regarding my treatment. Without my input he/she can't make positive decisions. Honest communications at its best!

You might be saying to yourself, "I don't have the time to write down everything, talk, listen and understand." Don't feel bad, you're not alone. If you feel overwhelmed, scared or nervous there is nothing wrong with taking someone close to you in the appointment room with you, in fact it's advised. As the saying goes, "Two heads are better than one." No doctor will object to you bringing someone along with you to ensure the communication lines between patient and doctor are successful. If they do well, you have another red flag to deal with.

Having someone else with you enables you to pay closer attention to what your doctor is telling you instead of worrying about what to write down. Some individuals, me included, have a tendency to concentrate more on ensuring that I get everything written down than having an open two-way communication with my doctor. This defeats the objective. If you have someone with you, then he/she is concentrating on getting everything on paper while you interact with your doctor. There are also other advantages to having someone with you. One advantage your companion can have by accompanying you is to eliminate the human nature aspect of the visit of holding back things you know you should tell your doctor but are scared of the diagnoses or treatments that might occur. Let's be honest, we all do it. Even if you write everything down on a note you still have to give it to the doctor. The majority of humans will go as long as they can without informing their doctors of things bothering them healthwise, especially men. We somehow think the pain will magically go away. It doesn't!

I've had several occasions where I've written my note but then before I go in to see the doctor I'll read over it and keep it in my pocket as opposed to giving it to the doctor. If the appointment is going good, then, unfortunately, I've kept some of the symptoms on the list to myself. Having someone with you eliminates the choice because they will ensure you give the note to the doctor or will bring up the symptom if you don't.

As always it still comes back to the patient having the ultimate responsibility because, as the patient, you have to ensure your companion knows of the symptoms in order to be effective. If the companion is your spouse or caregiver he/she probably already knows most of the symptoms and might even detect some the patient isn't aware of or doesn't want to admit. It's the responsibility of the companion to ensure all symptoms and responses to previous treatments are brought up during the appointment.

The companion must not be afraid of the patient's possible negative response to bringing up certain situations. Again before the appointment it might seem like a good idea to the patient to have a companion with him/her but when the time comes and fear creeps in he/she can have a change of mind. If you are the companion you have to be strong and not worry about the patient's initial reaction, but, instead, just keep focused on your responsibility of ensuring the doctor is informed regarding everything you know about the patient's health situation. As we will discuss later, being a caregiver can be hard but it's your primary responsibility to ensure your loved one gets the best health care possible. For that to happen you have to sometimes make the patient angry as you inform the doctor of things he/she, subconsciously or consciously, forgot to mention.

As the patient an important thing you must do to ensure the person, or persons, with whom you're comfortable with as a caregiver or companion is to make sure he/she is included as someone the doctor can give out and discuss your health with. In order for this to happen they must be included on your Health Insurance Portability and Accountability Act (HIPAA) Privacy Rule sheet you complete with each of your doctors. It should be included in the pile of paperwork you fill out the first time you see a doctor; if not ask for it. The HIPAA laws were implemented to protect the patient's health information from being given to just anyone and, legally, no medical professional is allowed to give out a person's health information except to those individuals listed on the patient's HIPAA sheet. So make sure any individual, such as your spouse, another family member, your caregiver or anyone else you're comfortable with, is listed with your doctor. This should not only be one of the first things you do but it should also be updated regularly as well. Note of caution, since the person will be able to have access to all of your health information make sure only those you trust are listed on your HIPAA sheet. Guard your health information closely because, not only is it personal, in the wrong hands it could cause you unnecessary and avoidable problems down the road as well. The HIPAA Privacy Rule is a good law. Let's make sure we use it as it was intended.

Another benefit of keeping things regarding your appointments, treatments, and results is the information can act as a log for you, and your doctors, to refer back to. How long should you keep the information? That's a decision for you to make based on your situation. If you use a computer with ample storage you could keep the information forever or save the data to an extended storage device such as a CD or USB storage device. However, it's a good idea to keep the information for a few appointments so you can see the progress of your treatments, especially if you have a chronic health condition.

Another thing you should do is keep a small notebook with information such as your health conditions, medications, insurance information, and any other vital information with you when you go to your appointments, especially to new doctors. Having this information available will not only help your doctor have a better understanding of your current and past health needs but will enable you to complete the necessary paperwork more efficiently as well. Having information in writing always outweighs your memory!

There's another responsibility you as the patient, or caregiver, has during your appointment other than insuring you've communicated all of your symptoms, reporting your activities since your last appointment, and having kept good documentation, and that's ensuring you ask the right questions. Once you've given the doctor all the information you can think of the ball is in your doctor's court to decide the diagnosis and treatments. However, it's still the patient's responsibility to ensure you understand what your doctor is suggesting you should do. As the patient, whose health is ultimately at stake, you must always be an activist and advocate for your own health and benefit rights.

If something doesn't seem right or feels wrong, never let it go without question. Do not under any circumstances fall into the stereotype myth that your doctor knows everything and you know nothing. In reality you have two distinct advantages over your doctor in regard to your health. The first, and most influential, is you know better than anyone (in fact you're the only ones who truly knows) exactly how you feel. As we stressed earlier, you must be in tune with your body because we are all unique individuals. Now is the time to put the knowledge of self to your benefit. Never let a doctor, or anyone else for that matter, tell you how you feel.

The second, and most powerful, advantage is your inner voice. If something is telling you your diagnosis or treatment isn't right, question it. Ask for details and explanations as to how and why these results were concluded. Ask for a second opinion or to see a specialist if your doctor hasn't already referred you to someone with more experience in this specific area of medicine. Listen, trust, and follow your inner voice.

You understand how your body is reacting and most likely how it will react to certain situations. My mother is a good example in contrast to myself. I can take pretty much any medications without negative reactions, prednisone being a good example. My mother, on the other hand, has trouble with pretty much any medication. Prednisone tears her up. So if a doctor just looks at medical cases and solutions, as opposed to listening with detail to the patient's unique circumstances and body makeup, the treatments will be the same with two very different results. However it's up to you, the patient, to ensure you have communicated how you feel and your concerns to your doctor or otherwise how will your doctor know?

Just so we're all on the same page, let's not confuse the feelings that something isn't right with this is something I don't want to do. There is a major difference here. Look at my case for a second. If I had known how to listen to my body, based on the diagnosis and failed treatments, and had trusted my inner voice as opposed to hearing what I wanted to hear even though I was aware I was being told the same thing over and over by those seven doctors during my pre-sarcoidosis diagnosis stage, then I would have advocated for myself by questioning the doctors and demanding to see a specialist. If I had advocated for myself at some point in those five years of runarounds I probably wouldn't be writing this book. That's a case of not reacting to my inner feelings that something just wasn't right because I didn't know, or want, to listen.

On the other hand I didn't want to take insulin and I fought it with every excuse I could. My endocrinologist kept telling me it was time, but I just straight up didn't want to start injecting myself. Even though my body was telling me it was time as my blood sugar readings were regularly in the 200 or over range, even in the morning when your blood sugar levels are at their lowest, and my inner voice was telling me it was time to do what I had to do in order to live a better quality of life, I refused to listen. That's a case of not reacting to my inner feelings simply because I didn't want to listen and out of fear.

The bottom line is your inner voice will lead you down the correct path if you learn to listen and follow. Don't let fear or intimidation stop you. Don't let lack of faith in yourself stop you. Don't put on blinders because you don't want to do what you have to do. Sometimes when our health care is concerned, it can be unpleasant, at first, and a lot of hassle. God made the human body to survive and with your inner strength along with your open, honest, and positive relationship with your doctor, regardless of the health condition, you can live a positive quality of life.

Work to build a positive relationship with your doctors. Take advantage of your appointment times and trust in your doctor's advice. But more importantly, trust in your inner voice to guide you and trust in your knowledge of yourself. As a team your quality of life will only improve!

...6...

Your appointment is your time to achieve the maximum benefits regarding your health and, in turn, will enable you to understand and achieve the maximum positive results from your doctor's diagnosis and treatments, and most of all will ensure you stay as healthy as possible. Use the time wisely!

7
Building A Medical Family

In today's medical environment it takes an entire family of medical professionals to treat a patient's medical needs. Your doctor might be considered the head of household but like all families there are other family members who have an impact on your life. Your medical family is no different.

Nurses are the first medical family members that come to mind. They play a more personal role in your medical life than any other medical professional, including your doctor. Nurses are, without a doubt, the most influential family members in regard to your medical experiences. Nurses are the backbone of the medical environment and always have been. It's the nurses with whom you will most often interface before and after you see your doctor or during any hospital visit. The majority of your preparation and follow-up will be done with the nurses. The importance of nurses cannot be underestimated, as they play a vital role in your medical treatment. Doctors could not possibly do his/her jobs without quality nurses to assist them!

Building and maintaining a positive relationship with your nurses is the most important relationship you will have. Unlike your doctor, who will probably be around for a while, your nurses could be here today and gone tomorrow, therefore causing you to start all over with the relationship building process just about the time everything is running smoothly. This reality in regard to helping keep quality nurses around is something that's out of the patient's hand, since we don't control the salaries, working hours or benefits…or is it?

In our current medical state, there's a serious shortage of good, quality nurses. In fact it's widely predicted that in ten years the shortage will be even greater, primarily due to the retirement of current nurses in the field. This is sad, not only because of being a registered nurse (RN) can be a rewarding job, both personally and financially, but also because most nurses are overworked which can be harmful to the patient. Maybe we as patients should take a more appreciative and proactive role in ensuring quality nurses feel appreciated in their roles and let them know how important they are to us. Quality/aware nurses can make a world of difference in regard to the positive quality of care a patient receives, and thus, in the successful recovery a patient has. Quality nurses have a major impact on your doctor's visit, hospital stay, emergency room visit or any other medical situation you might encounter because you can bet the farm a nurse will be the primary person taking care of you in all of those situations, regardless of where you might be or what's wrong with you.

There have been several issues reported as to why we can't seem to keep or attract quality nurses. Some are out of the patient's realm, such as being overworked. This comes from having too many patients per nurse, which again goes back to not being able to maintain or attract new nurses. Another issue widely reported is the lack of resources available to nurses so they can do their job effectively. Budget cuts and other financial issues have a major impact on this problem. Somehow the administrative branch of the medical community needs to come up with some type of solution. Isn't that supposedly why they get paid the big bucks?

Red tape causes a lot of the problems, but so does greed. Profit drives a lot of the decisions in our current medical state, not patient priority, which is what the medical community should be about. But reality is what it is and money is a major issue and requirement in order to ensure proper resources are in place. Where and how the money is spent is something patients do not control. Fact is even though the patient might not be able to do anything to make proper resources available, I suspect we will pay the price in the end, either with our health and/or our money. After all, it's always the consumer who pays for corporate problems, which is what today's medical facilities are.

Another problem reported and one we as patients must be held accountable for is rudeness from patients and their family members. This behavior is unacceptable! I understand in emergency room situations, patients are not themselves due to trauma. No one expects a patient suffering from a traumatic situation to be a jolly old soul. So understand that's not the situations being referring to. In life and death situations you, and your family members, must do what you have to do to survive! In those situations Mother Nature takes over for you and medical training takes over for the doctors and nurses. So let's skip over that scenario.

I also understand when you're sick or worried about your health's outcome your frame of mind is not what it should be. This is true for family members as well. However, that does not, under any circumstance, give any of us the right to use the nurses as a punching bag or stress ball. Being rude will not get you any better service and will not help your health situation. It will only cause friction and tension, thus causing undo stress in an already stressful situation. Worth repeating, no one expects a person to be in the best of moods during times of crisis or pain, but we're all still human and no one deserves to be treated with disrespect just because, for some reason, you feel the need to vent on someone. You must find another way to relieve your anxiety. Would you stay in a work environment where your customer constantly disrespects you? In the end we all suffer, so please, for us all, try to maintain respect towards, not only the nurses, but also everyone you come in contact with, even when you're sick.

On the flip side, if you're treated disrespectful, which also happens due to the stress levels and unqualified nurses feeling, for some reason, they can take their frustrations out on someone who is stuck in bed, report them immediately. When I said no one has the right to disrespect another person regardless of the situation that goes for everyone - patients, family members and medical professionals. There's absolutely no excuse for a medical professional to be disrespectful to a patient or family member - ever. Let me give you an example to backup this statement.

Both my mother-in-law and father were diagnosed with cancer and spent a lot of time in cancer centers both in Detroit, Michigan, and Tallahassee, Florida, receiving treatments. Not one time in all of our visits to either cancer center, and there were a lot of visits, did anyone show any attitude or disrespect to, not only them, but any other cancer patients being treated. Not one time, and there were situations where patients were throwing up on the nurses, family members were in depressed states of mind, people were given life altering news, exhaustion had set in from both a physical and mental standpoint on all parties involved and many other situations that causes normal people not to be themselves, was there ever a word, look (looks can be as disrespectful as anything else, sometimes even more so) or action of disrespect from any member of the medical staff, especially the nurses.

I promise you not only were these medical professionals over-worked but they also dealt with a lot of pressure in regard to the high emotional levels of cancer patients and their families. Each and every one of those nurses and other medical professionals stayed professional at all times. My point - if they can do it under those circumstances there's absolutely no reason whatsoever others can't do the same. No one was drafted into the medical profession and everyone understood ahead of time what was involved so do your job with respect.

Another problem patients cause, especially with female nurses, and something that's not mentioned very much publicly, is sexual harass-ment. The harassment ranges from the male patients constantly call-ing female nurses "sweetie or cutie" to sexual jokes to inappropriate touching. Most nurses chalk the harassment up to the excuse that the male patient doesn't feel good or is confused. Personally I feel the male patient just feels he can get away with it since he's "sick" or wants at-tention. Being in the hospital or sick doesn't give anyone any more of a right to make inappropriate remarks or take actions than any other part of society. Just because someone must deal with your body in private ways, like sponge bathing you because you can't bathe yourself, doesn't make it a welcomed sexual situation. It's the business of your health!

There's a very fine line between nurses meeting their professional responsibilities to a patient and protecting themselves. Fortunately few rape cases are reported. The bottom line is sexual harassment on any level causes additional tension among nurses and is something we as patients can eliminate. This applies to female patients actions toward male nurses as well. Just because you're a male nurse doesn't mean you want or are comfortable with female patients flirting with you. In to-day's world, same sex sexual harassment counts as well.

Maybe subliminally patients, family members and others feel its okay to let out their frustrations on nurses because of another widely mentioned cause of tension among nurses - a lack of respect. This, I just don't understand because being a nurse is an important and fulfilling occupation we as patients, family members and doctors, need. I don't know if it comes from the old timer mentality that portrays nurses as women who can't be doctors, and Lord knows, the respect level can be even less for male nurses, or if somehow nurses are just looked upon as a servant to the doctor.

I thought it was an interesting scene in the movie "Meet The Parents" where the future son-in-law (Ben Stiller) was a male nurse, even though he passed the medical exam with flying colors. At the breakfast table with the in-law family he was explaining to the two other doctors (the other future son-in-law and his father) he "wanted" to be a male nurse instead of a doctor. The reason was so he could deal with the patients and not all of the bureaucracy, but nobody believed him. They all made fun of him as they laughed, then just cut him off in the middle of his sentence as if he wasn't even talking, and definitely what he was saying wasn't important. I think that's a good example of the attitude toward most nurses, which is wrong!

If you saw the movie there was another scene at the beginning where he was helping a patient and the patient actually thought he was the doctor. In fact, in the follow-up movie "Meet The Fockers", at the beginning he actually delivers a baby as well. Later on there was a scene where the father-in-law was showing a baby learning cards, which included a female nurse figure, and he makes a sarcastic remark there were no male nurse cards, again as if being a male nurse, or nurse period, was not a respected job!

The next time you're at your doctor's office or in a hospital just pick out one nurse and watch them while you wait. I bet you will get worn out just watching everything they have to do. I can't stress enough the difference a quality nurse makes in today's medical environment since they seem to do a lot of what the doctors did several years back. Remember, it's the little things that make the big differences and every detail is important so let's ensure we give the good nurses incentives to stay in the nursing field. I can't think of many other occupations where the work can be so rewarding. There's absolutely no reason why anyone should not give a nurse the ultimate respect they deserve. We need them!

Nursing is one of the few fields where, not only getting a job, but also maintaining it, is wide open with no end of opportunities in sight. The opportunities are countless for qualified individuals. Not only are there opportunities from a normal career standpoint but also a lot of incentives other than a paycheck exist as well. There are even opportunities for what's termed "gypsy or traveling nurses" where you can work a temporary contract (say two or three years) and have your living expenses paid on top of your salary. These are very popular in areas where there's a state requirement which limits the ratio of patients to a nurse.

There are opportunities for others that reside outside the United States, such as Africa, Asia, Canada or the Middle East. Several programs exist where individuals come to this country and work as a nurse to get the experience, then after their two to three year commitments they return home. I think we should figure out a way to keep those qualified individuals on the job here after their required commitments are over as well. I understand quality nurses are needed worldwide, but since I live in America, I must say we need all of the qualified and experienced nurses we can get! So keep in mind the nursing field is not only one of the most important aspects of the medical environment but a golden employment opportunity as well.

As far as building your medical family here's some advice for you to remember. The first thing you do is go out of your way, even if you're not feeling very good, and get in good with the nurses. It's just like in the corporate world when you go to a new job the first person you get in good with is the secretary or administrator (whichever title they hold at your corporation). If you move into an apartment or condo the first person you get in good with are the maintenance people. Always get in good with the people who do the actual work because they're the ones who actually run the business. The medical environment is no different.

One important fact you have to remember, and we can never lose track of, when building your relationships with your nurses, or anyone else in the office for that matter, is you're dealing with a human being. Remember that the nurse is probably one who is overworked and is dealing with people who are either sick, frustrated, tired of waiting or just don't want to be there. It's amazing how far a little kindness and respect will get you!

This may sound simple and obvious. You may get tired of hearing it, but when you're sick the simple and obvious can easily be forgotten without realizing it unless it has been permanently drilled into your memory bank. Treating each other with respect is the most important element in building good relationships on any level, but it's only the beginning.

Honest, respectful communications will give any relationship a positive start. I know this is hard for someone who has had to wait for over an hour to just get in to see the doctor, but as you already knew, in this situation that's just sometimes how it is, so try your best to be respectful. It's not the nurse's fault so why use him/her to vent your frustration? Nurses see a lot of patients on a daily basis, but if you will just be respectful, you will stand out and like all human beings when you're treated with respect, respect is usually returned. Sometimes, like it or not, you have to go out of your way to get the relationship started on the right track. Never forget the bottom line - it's your health that's at stake here so always do what you have to do to get the most out of your situation. Building a positive relationship with the nurses you come in contact with will benefit you in more ways than you can begin to realize.

It doesn't hurt to show a little interest in their lives as well. Sometimes just listening with interest will go a lot farther than any words can take you. They have frustrations as well and a friendly, interested ear might just be what they need at the moment. Who knows, you might even find you actually enjoy the brief, but sincere, conversations you might engage in. When you stop and think about it, a doctor's visit, in a way, can be a kind of social visit because we all know any doctor's visit will take time, so try and make the best of it to the best of your ability. As we have already discussed, just don't waste your time or the medical professional's time once the appointment actually starts with your doctor. Use your time wisely and constructively but at the same time take the time to be friendly and respectful to those individuals you encounter, especially the nurses.

From a patient's perspective there's no one in the office you want on your side more than the nurse. I usually pick out the one nurse who seems to be the one everyone goes to or the one who seems to get things done and do all I can to get on their good side. Although it's important to build good relationships with all of the nurses, it's just as important to have one special primary contact with whom you're comfortable. Do keep one thing in mind though - don't take advantage of your relationship. Crying wolf will be the worst thing you can do because once you have the crying wolf reputation, your request will fall on deaf ears and will automatically drop to the bottom of the "To Do" list. Trust me, you don't want that label!

Nurses are the lifelines of the medical profession in regard to treating patients. Nurses perform so many procedures other than drawing blood or giving you an injection. Plus, wouldn't you rather have someone you're cool with sticking you with a needle than someone who thinks you're a jerk? Remember human nature!

We need our nurses so, as a patient, do your best to show every nurse the respect they deserve. Let them know you appreciate what they do for you. Maybe even take a look at your own life and see if the nursing field is for you. As an adult, you're never too young or too old to start a career in nursing and, at least for the immediate future, the opportunities will be waiting for you. For those already in the nursing fields remember, we as patients, really aren't ourselves and we need respect too. Together we can both achieve our goals - for the patient to get better healthwise and for the nurse the fulfilling reward of playing a major part in the healing process. Successful together. Isn't that really what relationships are all about?

There are a couple of other members of your medical family who have an impact on the care you receive and the stress levels you experience such as the medical assistants and billing clerks. Especially in today's medical environment, they both are extremely important and can't be avoided at some point in time.

The medical assistants, or as the term is used for the sake of this book, are those who perform duties other than the doctor or nurse in the physician's office and take care of the office work. Building and maintaining a positive relationship with them will make the process easier when you need to get required/routine tasks completed. There are the basic tasks of scheduling appointments, or better yet, scheduling appointments around your schedule. Depending on how good your relationship with them is will determine if they can pull any of those magical strings to get you in to see the doctor when there are no "known" appointments available, as most doctors keep a few slots open for emergency appointments. Being honest about your needs and relaying that information in a positive, calm tone makes a big difference in the response and results you get. Frustration plays a big part in their lives as well, as it does yours.

They too have probably been yelled at or spoken to in attitude more than once during their day, so a positive tone is probably a welcomed relief for them and will no doubt make a difference in their willingness to go the extra mile to accommodate your needs. In fact, a lot of them are probably tired from their other responsibilities outside the office such as school, training or supporting a family. The cycle of rudeness touches us all! Never forget, regardless of the profession or position we should always treat others as we want to be treated.

There are other advantages of building a positive relationship with the medical assistances. One will be when it comes to dealing with insurance referrals. Although a lot of insurance plans are now allowing you to see doctors within your network without a referral there are some who still require a referral in order to see a specific specialist. In fact some offices, although you don't need a referral, will require a letter from your primary doctor in order to see you.

You may also, as a result of your insurance requirements, need to have certain medical files, such as your last blood tests, faxed for your specialist's appointment. Referrals and other insurance requirements are just part of the medical process in our current times so as a patient you can use all the help you can get to make dealing with the process easier and more successful. Work on establishing a process with the medical assistant. Learn what information you need to provide them in order to have the proper documentation available for your appointment time. Establishing this process will ensure you get your information on time, thus your appointments and test will go on as planned. Always keep in mind this is a team effort. You can't do it alone so don't isolate yourself by not building a positive relationship with the entire medical staff.

Having a good relationship with the medical assistants will be of value when prescriptions are needed to be called in or responded to from your pharmacy. Understanding other office cost policies such as fees charged for filling out forms or getting copies of your medical records are duties for which the medical assistants are usually responsible. In fact some doctors are starting to charge an annual administration fee, in addition to your regular charges, as a result of the tremendous amount of numerous forms. So be aware! Billing issues are another area where having a positive relationship with your medical assistant will be of value as you must now also work with another family member - the billing clerk.

Building a relationship with the billing clerk is a little different than those others I've written about because usually the relationship you build with them will only (fingers crossed) happen on a one-time basis...the issue at hand. They can be like that long distant cousin you only see every few years, have a good time with or dread every moment, then they're out of your life until next time, whenever that may be. Sometimes the longer the better!

The most important factor in building this relationship, and getting positive results, is for you to stay calm and speak in a respectful tone at all times, regardless of how frustrated you might get, how many times you have to repeat yourself, how long you have to be on hold (this will happen a lot), how many clerks you're transferred to or how many questions you have to ask, sometimes more than once. Staying calm will allow the clerks to not get frustrated with your attitude and in the end most will go the extra mile to help you resolve your issue. Although it might not seem like it at the time, you will save time by just following the process and if you have to take it to another level or appeal you've already followed their processes so you're one step ahead of the game because that's the first thing you're going to be asked by the next level. If you haven't followed the correct process they'll send you right back and here you go again.

Another factor that's as important as staying calm and respectful is for you to have a good understanding of your insurance policy, what you had done and what you should be charged for. Being able to talk knowledgably about your policy and what you're entitled to from a benefit standpoint will automatically get you respect from the billing clerk. I can't tell you the number of times I've called regarding a billing issue and sensed an attitude in the clerk's tone as they talk down to me. I immediately find a tactful way to interject the fact I worked in the insurance industry supporting a health care claims system for over 16 years so I understand the behind the scenes processes that occur. Immediately I sense the attitude go away as if all of a sudden we're now on the same level in regard to knowledge of what's going on or else they feel they aren't going to be able to intimidate me or pull the wool over my eyes anymore. It might not sound fair but it's reality. Remember to do this in a calm and respectful way because no one likes for someone else to tell them how to do their job. Be tactful and suggestive as opposed to cocky and demanding, or else it will do more harm than good. Never lose track of the fact you're interacting with another human being who holds the key to your positive solution.

You didn't need to have worked in the insurance industry in order to get the same result. The same positive results can be achieved by letting the billing clerk know you understand your policy and what's being billed, especially if you have documentation to back it up such as an Explanation Of Benefits. You can never have too much documentation so keep everything for at least two years or know where you can obtain a copy if needed as a lot are available online.

Following up with what was discussed in a timely manner is critical as well. Pick your follow-up time wisely because you don't want to come across as a pest but instead come across as someone who holds others to their word, just as you keep yours. You don't want too much time to pass with the issue unresolved because then it's going to take more effort on your part to resolve the issue, and to be honest, sometimes that's what the billing departments want you to do - pay it, then forget about it. I don't think so!

Keep in mind at all times, although you need the assistance of the billing clerk and medical assistance to resolve billing issues, it is the patient's responsibility to do what is needed to get it resolved. Even if you don't feel you should have to do this or that, keep in mind you're responsible for the payment, right or wrong, so if it's wrong, get it corrected. Getting mad and yelling at the clerk might make you feel better (actually it will make you feel a lot better), but it will only hurt your chances of getting the issue resolved in a timely manner because you've now established yourself as a jerk in the eyes of the clerk. Who do you think they will go out of their way to help first, someone who has been respectful to them or a jerk? This is important to remember and practice because the fact is you can't go in and correct the system, only they can!

Respectfulness goes a long way in any relationship, especially ones where individuals are under a lot of stress and frustration. Having honest, knowledgeable and respectful communications lets everyone involved know what's expected of him/her without intimidation. Unfortunately intimidation is a common practice with some billing folks, especially when the issue gets complicated. Never be intimidated by a billing issue or anyone trying to deny you what you feel you rightfully deserve in any circumstance or situation in your life. Never!

Although I could give you examples I've experienced many times over, let me give you one where it shows how advocating for yourself and not being intimidated allows you to get not only positive results but also what you're entitled to. This example is in regard to an oral surgery I had to remove a tooth that had been causing problems for a long time and there was nothing else we could do to save it. When I went for my initial consultation I was impressed by the respect and knowledge the surgeon had for not only sarcoidosis but also for the various secondary conditions and medications I was under. He agreed we needed to extract the tooth (my left bottom back tooth or #18) and with everything I had going on healthwise he would need to sedate me as well. In addition, anytime I must be put under sedation my endocrinologist requires I be given 100MGs of hydrocortisone while the procedure is being performed. The surgeon agreed with this requirement and wanted me to contact my endocrinologist to get any additional instructions. As always, my prednisone was increased the day of the surgery then slowly decreased over the course of the next few weeks until I was back to my normal dosage. The surgeon also prescribed medications to take starting a couple of days before the surgery. I was pleased with the process and attention to detail so far, but then came his billing department.

As the medical assistant was setting up my appointment, I learned it was going to be several weeks before she could get me in. Since I was in constant pain and she wasn't hearing anything I was trying to explain to her, I had her page the surgeon who told her to book me within a week at his other office (he shared his time between two offices) because I needed this tooth extracted as soon as possible because of other health issues. She didn't seem too happy about adjusting her scheduling but did anyway and was able to get me in the Monday after next (it was currently Thursday). She then wrote up my estimate that turned out to be $365. This immediately raised a red flag because since I knew I was going to need dental work (in fact this was the primary reason I waited so long) we had purchased through my wife's employer the top of the line dental coverage that covered everything at 80 or 100% and this total wasn't close to 80% based on the total pre-insurance cost she had provided.

When I questioned my cost I was told the extraction was covered at 80%, however; due to the long standing policy of the dental insurance company, if you're not getting a minimum of two teeth surgically extracted then the IV sedation is not covered and I would be responsible for 100% of the cost ($250). In addition the hydrocortisone was not covered and again I would be responsible for 100% of the cost ($75). I told her this didn't seem right and could she verify it. She gave me a sour look (maybe because it was 5:00 P.M. on a Thursday afternoon and she had already had to adjust her schedule for me), picked up the phone and must have called another billing clerk in the office because all she said on the phone was, "When less than two teeth are extracted then the IV sedation is not covered, right? That's what I told him." She hung up and said, "I was right (with a smirk on her face) it's not covered and it never has been so you're responsible." She reminded me of an elementary school child taunting another child on the playground. I just looked at her with a chuckle (which probably ticked her off even more) and said, "Okay".

I had been in these conversations before and wasn't going to waste my time with someone who had an attitude, plus no authority anyway. I went to pay my $5 office visit co-pay but she didn't had change for a $20 bill so she told me to just pay it when I have the surgery. The next week they sent me a bill anyway with a handwritten note attached reminding me I forgot to pay my co-pay at the time of the visit, when it was required, and I needed to submit it as soon as possible. I sent a $5 check with a handwritten note of my own. You can use your imagination regarding what I wrote, as I had a feeling this was going to be a long adventure and I wanted them to understand you can't intimidate me with handwritten notes!

The next morning I called the insurance company myself and explained the situation. Turns out the two-tooth minimum is a longstanding policy that still makes no logical sense to me. Do they feel you should be able to withstand the pain of one tooth but not two? Anyway, I knew there are always exceptions and I asked if a review of my claim could be done. The insurance associate with the insurance company was very helpful and understanding as she said, "That was just what I was going to suggest." So I had the surgeon's office fax over the proposed bill along with the written information regarding my current health condition and medications I had provided them during my appointment to the insurance company. I followed-up with the insurance company to ensure they had received the fax. Then, as is so common, I waited patiently.

I followed-up again the next Thursday and left a voice message with the insurance associate I was dealing with. On Friday I received a return call from her. After reviewing my case it was agreed the IV sedation should be covered at 80%, therefore the allowed amount was now $219 and the coverage was $186.15 while I paid only $32.85. However, the hydrocortisone was not going to be covered and I would be responsible for the $75 cost. A Pre-Authorization Explanation Of Benefits would be sent out to the surgeon's office and a copy to myself that same day. Overall I was happy and on Monday I paid my new cost of $125 as opposed to the original $365. The surgery went perfectly, I started feeling better overall healthwise and it was a successful experience, or so I thought.

In a few weeks I received a bill from the surgeon's office for $186.15 and another handwritten note requesting I pay this amount in a timely manner. I tried calling but got a voice mail so I left my name, number and the reason for my call. I also replied with a letter stating my insurance company covered this cost and they received a Pre-Authorization Explanation Of Benefits explaining this (how else would they have known not to charge me at the time of service?) and I included a copy of mine just in case they had lost theirs. I also had just moved so I gave them my new address and phone number if they had any questions. I never heard back from my voice mail. Again, I thought that was the end of it but was wrong.

In another few weeks I received another bill with a stronger worded handwritten note, this time telling me to send in my payment within seven days or else other action would be taken, in all capital letters. It was obvious they had not done anything with my reply; in fact the bill had been forwarded from my old address once again, which proved my point. I knew what the problem was so I called the insurance company myself, told them the situation then asked what type of claim form had been sent in? Sure enough, the surgeon's office had sent in what's called an "In-For-Pay" claim form as opposed to a "Pre-Authorization" claim form, which should have been sent in based on the Pre-Authorization Explanation Of Benefits they had received. The insurance associate made the adjustment to the claim right then so a payment would be sent to the surgeon's office and told me to please inform the surgeon's office they do not need to do anything because we have done their job and taken care of it for them. You could hear the frustration in her voice towards the surgeon's staff as she thanked me for following up and understanding the process. In fact she jokingly suggested I go to work for the surgeon's office myself.

I replied to the surgeon's office with another letter (after I left another message on their voice mail that, too, was never returned) explaining the situation and that we had taken care of it for them and they need not do anything. Also I sent a copy of everything to the surgeon making sure to include the letters sent to me with the attempted intimating remarks. I felt it was important to let the doctor know of the unnecessary hassle and attempted intimidation his staff was using when the reality is they didn't do their job correctly. If he wanted he could address the way (with proof) his staff was performing and the customer service they were providing. After all in the end it reflected on him. In a few days I received another Explanation Of Benefits from my insurance company stating the $186.15 had been paid and, of course, I never heard from the surgeon's office again and would be reluctant to return, if needed. Customer service really does matter!!!

This is a perfect example of not taking the first quote you receive when you feel it's not right and never pay a bill you know is not right just because there are intimidating remarks written on it, even if they are personal and handwritten. Attempted intimidation doesn't make a wrong situation right but is a more common practice than you might think. Having a good understanding of the process and having a positive relationship with the medical assistants, nurses and doctors can help tremendously when these situations arise, especially when the billing is done offsite, which is a common practice. I can't stress it enough, having positive relationships with your medical family and understanding the processes are a necessity in today's medical environment in ways you'll never imagine until the situation is upon you. It might then be too late!

Now if you've tried to build a positive relationship with members of your medical family and you're still having problems, you must take action to correct the problem. It's just good relations for you to do what you should as a human being to build a positive relationship, but, the fact is, some people are just jerks and some in the medical profession are in the business strictly for a profit. In the medical field there's no room for jerks or greed because the bottom line is they're there to perform a job. Regardless of the situation, you, the patient, are their customer. Customer service is something we seem to lose track of in America these days but customer service is still a requirement for any profession that serves other people, regardless if it's in the retail, restaurant, hotel or medical profession.

Over the many years I've spent as a chronic patient, I've seen and experienced it all, from the positive to the down right disrespectful. If you feel you've done all you can to build a positive relationship with your doctor's staff and they treat you with disrespect or do not follow-up on their job responsibilities, do the following: let the doctors know (as I did in my intimidation example with the oral surgeon), because unless you tell them they probably don't know what's going on outside of your visit with them. Most doctors in private practice hire their own staff, but in medical facilities it's usually the facilities that provide staff to the doctor. Either way if a staff member isn't doing his/her job the doctor can, and should, take action to correct the problem. If he/she doesn't take action and nothing changes you might want to consider changing doctors. There are too many good doctors with professional staffs available to stay with a doctor and be disrespected. After all the majority of your time is spent with the staff. It could keep you from actually going to the doctor as you should and if that happens your quality of health has been impacted as well and you just can't allow that to happen. Plus, I guarantee you if enough patients leave a doctor then he/she will correct the problem because regardless of how dedicated anyone is to his/her profession, unless you're a volunteer, you're working for money.

I want to give you something to think about I've learned primarily from my mother and mother-in-law, as well as from my wife, that will help build not only your medical family relationships but all of those other relationships in your life as well. The first thing is never hesitate to do something special for someone, especially if they do something for you, even if you feel it was something they should have done or it's their job. If you're like me, and I'm not proud to admit this fact about myself, this thoughtful action is something that slips my mind most times, even though I may have the intention.

My mother makes the best chocolate pies. Whenever someone does something kind for her or our family, she usually bakes them a pie in gratitude. Even when the logic behind the gesture seems odd when you think about it. For example, when my father was first put in home hospice neighbors and friends would bring my mother and father food so they wouldn't have to cook or go out to eat. In return my mother baked some chocolate pies to give back in return, therefore she ended up cooking anyway. But she felt giving back was the right thing to do and she was correct.

That same logic helps build a strong relationship with your medical family as well. It doesn't hurt to bake them something or bring them something to eat from time to time. As we have said many times, they're human and humans love to be appreciated in caring, personal ways. How many times have you thought to do this or seen other patients do such kind and thoughtful acts? I bet not many, if any.

I've overheard a few conversations (and I stress "few") in the doctor's office where a patient or family member of a patient called and told the staff they were bringing something special in the next time they come. The staff member would get off the phone with a big smile on his/her face and everyone would comment when told of the upcoming treat as you could just feel their spirits go up a level. If cooking isn't your thing, then recognize them with something you made or are interested in, even if it's just gift certificates or a dozen donuts (well maybe a healthier snack would be appropriate in this situation). Now you might say you spend enough money with them as it is, you just don't have the time or better yet, like I mistakenly/selfishly tell myself, they're just doing their job. But think of it this way. There are many things you can do that don't cost anything or take much effort on your part. How would it make you feel if someone did the same for you? Plus from a health standpoint, giving is one of the best therapies there is. Try it sometime.

The other thing I learned was from my mother-in-law. Her thing was sending cards. Regardless of the occasion, be it a holiday, special occasion, thank you, get well or "just because", she always made it a point to send cards. After her death we started noticing how much of a positive effect her cards had on those who received them. Almost everyone who knew her mentioned her cards and some even had saved them from years back. The impact of her thoughtfulness and efforts were noticed, even if the gesture seemed minor. To those receiving one of her cards, especially when not expected, truly brighten their day and life. The same holds true for your medical family. They deal with enough rudeness and lack of thoughtfulness that I guarantee you a simply "Thank You" is a welcomed gesture. To receive a card on a special day or just to hear "Thank you for your support" will go a long way in building a positive relationship.

Oh, as for my wife. Well, she does both and then some. Those three thoughtful unselfish women have taught me it's the little acts of kindness and appreciation that mean the most in relationships, regardless of the level the relationship is on. Your medical family will appreciate sincere acts of kindness from you, and in return, your relationships and success of your health will only improve. What do you have to lose?

...7...

All relationships, personal, professional, and medical, have the same basic requirements in order to be successful. I strongly believe if everyone would only follow, to the best of his/her ability, the golden rule of "Treat others as you want to be treated" then our relationships would blossom. Can you imagine how beautiful this world would be if we took the time and consideration to treat others with respect?

8

Dental And Pharmaceutical Connections

There are two more members of your medical family that are sometimes excluded when you consider those who ensure you maintain a healthy quality of life but in reality are as important and can have as much of a dramatic impact on your health as any medical professional we have already discussed. Building positive relationships and using both as a constant resource are vital to your overall health. Like a favorite aunt or uncle these two members of your medical family deserve special attention.

First is your dentist. Never put off dental work or take it lightly because it will, in time, have a negative impact on other health issues. When I was experiencing the tooth problem I described in my previous billing example I started experiencing other health issues as well. I was always tired and was finding my overall health declining as little things were starting to pop up. As soon as the tooth was removed my health returned to "normal" before any major issues developed.

When you have dental problems the bacterium can get into your blood stream and travel freely throughout your body. For me that's a problem for a couple of reasons. Due to sarcoidosis my immune system is abnormal and doesn't react in a normal way, without additional prednisone. When a bacterium enters my body it can cause problems. To add to the problem, being a diabetic, when bacteria or viruses enter my body they will find the weakest area and attack. This is why some diabetics can have something wrong in one area of their body, then another area that was already weak gets worse. Bacteria from your decaying teeth or gums, already in your bloodstream with the freedom to travel at will, is not a good thing and will do you damage unless you do something about it via medication, or better yet, get the problem corrected by your dentist.

Another issue when you're experiencing pain in your teeth or gums is you won't eat appropriately and we all know lack of a proper diet can cause numerous health issues. Letting pain go for a long period of time, in your mouth or any other part of your body, only increases the chances you're going to experience other health problems. Pain is the most obvious way your body warns you something is wrong. If I had reacted when my tooth first started hurting and not waiting until the pain was constant and too much to handle, I probably would still have tooth #18 in my mouth.

Another good way to tell something is wrong from a dental perspective is a new case of bad breath. A different body odor is a warning sign, possibly before the pain actually starts. As a caregiver you might find it awkward to tell the patient that he/she needs to address this issue. I once had a tooth I knew was causing problems but I didn't realize it was so obvious by way of my breath until my wife told me. Like body odor sometimes you don't notice your own odor. You should however notice if you rub your finger on your gums if there is an odor or on your toothbrush. If so then you have something you need to address. Go see your dentist! Now!

Going to the dentist seems to scare most of us even more than having surgery. Why? I know I have some really messed up memories of my dentist visits as a child. Our dentist was located above the Emporium department store and if I remember right you would walk up these creepy wooden stairs. This I remember for a fact - you would sit in the waiting room and listen to the drill being used on the patients ahead of you. Back then (1960s), at least at this dentist, he didn't use Novocain on children when filling a cavity. As a result I remember to this day the sound of the drill "was" as bad as the pain associated with it. I was scared to death to go the dentist and unless the pain in my mouth was just too much to hide I didn't dare say my teeth bothered me. I think a lot of us have that mental concept when the word "dentist" comes to ear and unjustly so, in today's modern era.

Fortunately the dental field has come a long way since the 1960s and the reality is dental work is not that painful, especially when you compare it to the pain and health problems you're going to experience if you don't make, and keep, your dental appointment. Your first step to good dental care is finding the right dentist. For those who don't have a family dentist, there are several ways to find a good one. Of course a personal referral is a good start but again when taking a referral make sure the person has used the dentist in the same manner in which you're planning to use him/her, same as with a doctor. There are several resources you can call to have a dentist recommended for you, as we discussed in finding a good doctor. Keep in mind the dentist usually must belong to the organization before they will refer them so you might want to learn what qualifications are required to join the organization. If just paying a fee is all it takes you might as well use the yellow pages since that's all it takes to advertise in them too.

As always your insurance company can be a resource as well, especially since your dentist needs to accept your coverage to gain full benefits and not cause you debt. Personally I wouldn't put too much emphasis on being close to your home or work since you shouldn't have to visit them that often, just regularly, but that's just personal opinion. I actually found my dentist I've had since 1992 through a free coupon, just like I did the chiropractor back in 1990, another subliminal example of God guiding my life. The important thing is to find a dentist you're comfortable with and even more important - use them. Food for thought…based on information I've heard from advertising for dental care, the majority of people over 65 years old have no teeth! I know my father was one of those individuals. I remember the pain he use to be in when he got the last ones removed and the hassles he would have with his dentures. This didn't happen overnight. Don't let it happen to you!

The same points go for building your relationship with your dentist and staff that go with your other medical family. Open communications, honesty, trust, and being comfortable all play major factors in your relationship, which in turn builds mutual respect. You must make sure, especially if you have chronic health conditions, you're honest about all of your health conditions and keep your complete health condition updated at your dentist's office. Don't think because you have diabetes, hypertension or take specific medications your dentist shouldn't be aware. Everything in your body affects everything in your body and your dental health is a major part of the equation. In my case the diabetes insipidus causes me problems due to not producing the proper amount of saliva at all times therefore my mouth gets dry and my teeth brittle. As a result of my diabetes mellitus if I want my teeth whitened I must use the two-week nightly process as opposed to the onetime treatment due to the possibility of easy infection of the gums. I also grind my teeth during my sleep as a result of the pain and muscle cramps I experience. Like the bad tooth problem I had was causing other health problems, other health problems can cause dental problems as well. When your body and health is concerned, what goes around comes around! Pay special detail to everything and let your doctor and dentist be the judge of what's important, not you the patient.

There are some health issues that can cause a person to be extremely sensitive to pain, especially in their teeth and gums. I know of several sarcoidosis patients for whatever reasons have a very hard time with their teeth. By making their dentist aware of this problem the dentist could take extra steps to ensure the procedures do not take a toll on the patient. For me, I have a hard time keeping my mouth open for any length of time due to the fact I'll get cramps in my jaws. Whenever I'm having work done where my mouth will need to be opened wide for my dentist to work, such as a root canal or preparing for a crown, especially if it's a back tooth, he will provide me with a bite block to help ease the cramps. A bite block is a simple device that goes between your teeth for you to bite on and thus keeps your mouth open. This simple process keeps me from having jaw cramps as often since I don't have to force myself to keep my mouth open but can relax by biting the device. In turn it helps my dentist work more effectively and in a timely manner because my mouth is opened in the manner he needs it. A simple win-win situation for everyone involved resulting from honest communications and understanding between my dentist and me.

To ensure I keep my dentist informed of my health conditions I constantly provide him with a document that includes my updated medications and health statuses to keep in my file. In fact they have a big red medical alert tag on my file, which makes me feel comfortable. I've actually found that be it my dentist, oral surgeon or periodontist, they seem to take my sarcoidosis more serious than other specialist in the medical field with which I have dealt and have gone so far as to do research on their own to get a better understanding, which is evident when I return for my next visit and they have new-found knowledge of the effect sarcoidosis has on my dental health. This has happened on more than one occasion and I've heard the same from other sarcoidosis patients. Maybe dentist don't have the same false ego as some in the medical field who seem to feel that since it's a medical health issue they should know everything about it or else they look stupid. In reality it's these doctors who obviously don't know enough about sarcoidosis, but pretend they do by throwing confusing medical terms at you; who are the ones that really look stupid and are too stupid to even realize it. Sometimes feigned intelligence is really stupidity. Honesty will always keep you on the right path.

You must be comfortable enough with your dentist, as with all your medical professionals, to discuss financial issues. This is even more important than with your medical doctor because your dental insurance is usually separate from your health care coverage and, in most cases, gives you a limit on the amount you can spend during a year before you're 100% responsible for the fees. Understanding this helps you both develop a dental plan for the year based on the seriousness of the problems and the financial end of your coverage, of course barring any emergencies. You must always look at the overall picture and be financially aware.

I had a tooth crack in 2005 (the one causing bad breath) to the point I needed what's called a crown extension by a periodontist. This is where your gum is cut back to expose more of the tooth before a crown could be applied or attached. It was June at the time and I only had enough money left on my 2005 limit to cover one of the procedures. So we came up with a plan based on the seriousness of the crack and impact on my other health issues where I could wait until October to get the crown extension. Then in 2006 when my limit started over and just when the crown extension should have healed I could get the crown. In the meantime I used a lot of mouthwash and mints. On January 2, 2006, at 8:00 A.M. I was the first dental patient of the New Year and everything worked out fine. By discussing my options openly and developing a plan, I received successful results both from a health and financial standpoint. Without a positive open relationship and an understanding of my insurance coverage beforehand, this never would have happened!

Don't take your dental health lightly and treat your dentist relationship as importantly as any other medical relationship. Dental work is really not what it was in the past but the result of not taking care of your teeth is. Just like you only have one body, you only have one set of teeth. Treat your dental health with the respect it deserves and make sure your dentist is an important part of your medical family and not just a picture of a distant relative in the family photo album.

Next is your pharmacist, a vital member of your medical family, if there ever was one. In fact, if you're like me and take a multitude of medications your pharmacist is more than a vital member of your medical family but is more like a resource which you and I can't do without. There are so many areas in which your pharmacist affects your life.

Personally, I strongly believe you should only use one specific pharmacy for your medication needs, if possible, especially if you have a chronic health condition and rely on your medications to survive. You can pick your pharmacy based on several personal factors such as location, insurance acceptance, price or discounts, knowledgeable pharmacists, online services, pharmacy hours, quality customer service, etc. There are so many options today including pharmacy chains, ma and pa neighborhood pharmacies, pharmacies in major super or discount stores, online pharmacies, medical center pharmacies (especially if you can obtain a discount with your insurance company that might be associated with the medical center), home delivery pharmacies and a variety of pharmacies setup in other locations such as grocery store chains. Your choices are many so take your time and find the pharmacy that fits your individual needs as you might receive a specific discount, such as my wife does with her medical center pharmacy, which we now use and save monies each time we fill a prescription, plus they have a wonderful staff as well. Look at all of your options. Once you have made your choice, its time to start building a lasting relationship because your pharmacist is more than someone who just fills a prescription, especially if you take multiple medications; he/she also plays a major part in your quality of life and is a good check and balance resource as well.

The most important factor in using the same pharmacy is they have all of your medications on file or online in one location accessible each time you get a new prescription or refill. There are many drugs that cause negative reactions if taken together. Even if you tell your doctor everything going on with you, including all of the medications you take, there are times when mistakes are made, especially if you're seeing a specialist as well. This is one reason why I keep stressing the importance of providing any new doctor, including your dentist, with an updated copy of the medications you're currently taking and why. A simple pain pill could cause a deadly reaction if taken together with another type of medication you might already be using. However using the same pharmacy, with all of the prescription medications you're on logged in their system, a red flag will show up if two drugs interact negatively with each other. Checks and balances are critical in all areas of your life but when it comes to prescription drugs - it could save your life. Once the red flag is raised you can go back to your doctor to ensure they meant for you to take this medication along with your other medications. Maybe they did, and then again, maybe they either overlooked it or you didn't inform them of the other medication. Either way, using the same pharmacy will just add another checkpoint to ensure your medications help you instead of sending you to the emergency room or worse yet - kill you.

Once you've established a pharmacy make it a point to interact with the pharmacy staff, especially the pharmacists, in order to build a positive relationship with them. Your pharmacist can help you get a better understanding of what to expect from a specific drug or give you options as far as generic version versus brand name medications. Most insurance policies require you use a generic drug, if available, but not all generic drugs are the same as the brand name. Basically a generic drug becomes available once the patent runs out, allowing others to use the formula. However there can be differences in the other parts of the formula other than the active ingredient, causing your body not to accept the generic version the same as it does the brand name. DDAVP, the nasal spray used to control my diabetes insipidus, is a perfect example for me. My body doesn't accept the generic version the same as the brand name, in fact the generic version stops working faster causing me to use more. There is also a noticeable difference in the two. With the generic version available to me, it must be kept in the refrigerator while the brand name can be kept at room temperature. Even for a non-pharmacist like myself, there's obviously a difference (maybe minor but still enough to cause me problems) between the two. I had to appeal to my insurance company a couple of times to be able to use the brand name without paying a penalty. I won both appeals with the help of my doctor and pharmacist.

Your pharmacists can also help you with other insurance issues. If you have a good relationship with them they will have no problem calling your insurance company when problems arise. In addition they can give you advice on how you might save money based on your coverage. Some drugs might be cheaper to buy outright than buying the approved amount and paying your co-pay (prednisone is a prime example). Other ways to help you maximize your financial burdens is to have your doctor write a larger quantity than the one-month quantity for a prescription. Most policies give you a one-month supply but on some drugs they will allow a three-month supply. The worst that can happen is you're denied and only given a one-month supply. The benefit of this process is you don't pay your co-pay as often thus saving you out-of-pocket money, especially on drugs you will take over a long period of time.

Writing the dosage as "take as directed" can sometimes allow you to get extra quantities as well. Be careful with this option as some pharmacies will assume "take as directed" to mean the minimum. I had this happen to me once when a the pharmacist "assumed" my prednisone prescription written as "take as directed with a quantity of 100 tablets" to mean one pill a day as opposed to the two pills a day and additional pills when problems occur, without contacting me or my doctor who wrote the prescription. When I went to have the prescription refilled I was unable to do so because I hadn't used up the approved amount of pills, based on the pharmacist's assumption. Needless to say this was a problem.

A couple of other ways your doctor can save you money on prescription drugs is to give you samples the drug company representatives leave with them, especially for a new prescription. They want the doctor to give them out so in the end the doctor will prescribe them instead of a competitor's. Don't expect your pharmacist to tell you that tip though, as most pharmacist don't care for the practice because it cost them business. Like all other aspects of the medical profession, pharmacies are in the business to make a profit as well. A message to the pharmacist, don't get mad at the doctors, they're just looking out for their patients and don't get mad at the patients because they're just trying to save money. After all if they don't give them out to their patients who need them from a financial standpoint they'll just go to waste. Some drug companies offer programs to help individuals who can't afford medications or don't have insurance coverage to obtain their drugs. Your doctor can assist you with these programs. Make it a point to ask.

When it comes to medications your pharmacist is the expert on prescription and nonprescription drugs. Use the resource often! Ask them, not only what to expect from a medication, but is there a non-prescription medication that might do the same. Do keep in mind your pharmacist is not your doctor so he/she cannot diagnose your condition, treatment or know all your medical history. However they do know your medication history (if you use a single pharmacy) and in turn can give you educated advice on your medications. Always consult your doctor if you decide not to take the prescribed medication or if you start taking something without a prescription. Nonprescription medications or even vitamins can cause reactions with other medica-tions. Always read the labels and never take anything before consulting with your doctor you aren't absolutely sure will not cause you harm or negatively interact with any other medications - **never**!

Understanding your medications is something you must take upon yourself to do as well. Your doctor is the first resource with your phar-macist being the second. You can also do research on the Internet, read required material that comes with every medication or buy one of the many books available that gives a variety of information regarding medications. I personally use a resource book that's updated every year and contains almost every drug there is by H. Winter Griffith, M.D. entitled *"Complete Guide to Prescription & Nonprescription Drugs"*. The book gives everything from brand name and generic versions to uses to dosage information to possible adverse reactions to possible interactions with other drugs and even possible interactions with other substances including those "other" drugs we might not tell our doctor about like marijuana, cocaine or alcohol. I usually buy an updated version every two to three years. (*NOTE...I have no affiliation with this author or book other than I have used it for years as a personal resource for the many different medications I use and personally feel it's worth recommending*).

I must warn you even though there's a lot of good information available, you need to be careful and as always understand the source before you take it to heart. Good examples are the many drug studies you hear about. Understand who funded them and who benefits from the findings. Understand within the material you receive all side effects must be listed so don't let that information scare you off. Be very careful of information on the Internet, for reasons we've already discussed. Be extra careful of SPAM, those e-mails you receive trying to get you to order medications at a cheap price online. If someone can't contact you upfront without trying to trick you to open the e-mail, or have to use trick subject titles, or steal someone else's address (I once had a spammer steal my website address as info@gilbertbarrjr.com to send out spam until I blocked the ability to steal an e-mail address), or not be able to give you sources to which you're able to reply to the e-mail without going to a web site or the address is undeliverable, delete the e-mail and report it as SPAM. If I had a dollar for every SPAM e-mail I get wanting me to use a specific drug or order a discount medication, I would be a billionaire. Yep, "If it's too good too be true then it probably is!" With medications it can also be deadly!

There are a lot of natural herbs available as well that claim will help you more than any prescription medication without the side effects. The same rules apply here. Understand the source, what research has been done and how they approach you. If someone can't come to you straight and be open about what they're selling, what you can expect or aren't available for questions, run away fast! Unfortunately a lot of people will prey on individuals who feel hopeless or desperate for a fast cure. I see it all the time with sarcoidosis patients. Since there's currently no cure for sarcoidosis and prednisone, a primary drug in treating the symptoms relating to sarcoidosis, has such a dramatic effect on a lot of patients, there are opportunists waiting around every corner to give you the miracle cure, for a discount price. Always consult your doctor and pharmacist regarding any medications you're considering and never be pressured into taking anything out of fear or false hope. As always the responsibility and consequences falls back on you, the patient.

There are several other things you, the patient, can do to help ensure your medication does what it's prescribed to do. The most important is to take it as prescribed. Since you already trust your doctor's judgment you must take the medication the way it was intended for you to take it. If it doesn't work correctly in regard to treating your condition or you have an adverse side effect, let your doctor know immediately. This is the only way you're going to know if a medication works or not.

Learning the side effects, even for those medications you take on a regular basis, is important to your quality of life. All medications have different effects on different people so you must understand how the medication affects you personally. Some of us can take medications without any problems while others have a fit, even in the same family, as evident between my mother and me. Never plan on doing anything out of the norm when you first take a medication until you understand how it makes you feel, especially something that could put you in danger like driving alone. Common sense plays a role here but there are times when common sense seems to be lost on us all. We all seem to think it won't happen to us. In regard to prescription medications learn your reactions, before you put yourself in possible harms way.

Another thing that's important for you to do is learn what your medications look like. Sounds simple but it can save your life. Learn the size and color of each medication you take. If you get a medication that doesn't look like it should, question it with your pharmacist immediately, before you take it. Don't rely on what the bottle or label says, go by what the medication looks like. If you were switched to a generic version that looks different, don't trust the bottle, ask your pharmacist. After all, even pharmacists make mistakes and the wrong medication could have slipped into your bottle by mistake or you were given someone else's prescription. Maybe it's only a generic version or even a different generic brand and everything is okay. Maybe your doctor called in a replacement due to the pharmacy being out of your normal medication. Maybe the drug company came out with a different design. Maybe your insurance rejected the normal medication because they want you to take this brand, an extremely common practice that can occur in the middle of your calendar year. Regardless, verify with your pharmacist "before" you take the medication not "after" you're in the emergency room with a deadly reaction. If your relationship with your pharmacist isn't strong enough to ask questions or no one is available at your pharmacy for questions, you have the wrong pharmacy.

Now if you don't accept my logic regarding using only one specific pharmacy, for whatever reason, make it a priority to let each pharmacy know all the medications you take, just like you do with your doctors.

Keeping everyone on the same page could save your life. Unless you're hooked on your prescription drugs and going from pharmacy to pharmacy and doctor to doctor so you can get prescriptions written and filled, you have no reason not to keep everyone on the same page. If you are hooked and using various pharmacies for that reason - please get help now!

It's easy to get addicted to prescription drugs and nothing to be ashamed of. Parents and grandparents, make sure your prescription drugs are not disappearing, getting spilled, refills missing or lost, and if they are address it with your children, especially your teenagers. Today's youth (or routinely referred to as Generation Rx) are getting hooked on their parents and grandparents' prescription drugs at an alarming rate, no different than adults. Don't be naïve and if anyone you know, including yourself is hooked on prescription drugs, for your own sake and the sake of those close to you, seek help immediately before you become a funeral!

In addition don't keep your prescription medications in your bathroom medicine cabinet but instead in a safe place close to your bed or on a high shelve out of normal reach. Believe it or not, others will look in your medicine cabinet while in your bathroom and if they're addicted to prescription medication, the temptation will be too much, so be safe. That way it won't be as easy for those in your household or friends visiting to sneak any of your prescription medications. If your prescriptions seem to run out a little early let it be a sign someone is hitting your bottle. People hooked on prescription drugs have the same habits as crack heads, only not as obvious, and we all have heard those stories!

It's also a good idea to keep a couple days supply of your medications in your car, along with a bottle of water, in case you're stranded and can't get home. When you travel always keep your medications on you and not in your luggage because you might get separated from your luggage, especially if you're flying. Another home tip is to have a safe bag with at least a week supply of your medications, a document with your health information including medication refill numbers along with the pharmacy telephone number and a few bottles of water available in case of an emergency such as a house fire. You can never be too prepared when it comes to your health because if you're like me, just a few days without my medications and I will be in serious trouble, if not dead! You can ask your doctor and pharmacist for any other advice on how to prepare healthwise for any emergencies. Prescriptions medications, your doctor and pharmacist are supposed to help you, not harm you, so use all three intelligently.

Here are a couple of last tips. First always check the expiration dates on your medications. Some people will keep their medications, and food, past their expiration dates because of distrust with corporate America, as they feel corporations just want them to buy more and the product is still good after the date. Personally I don't take a chance with my food and especially with my medications. I just make sure I don't buy too much so I can use the food or medications up before they expire. If your medications do expire make sure you get rid of them in a safe manner like flushing your pills down the toilet so they don't fall into the wrong hands. "Better safe than sorry!"

The second thing is to check to see if you can write off your medications, along with other medical expenses, on your tax returns. Your pharmacy can provide you with documentation at year's end that will give you the total amount of prescription medications you used during the year so you don't have to worry about keeping all of your receipts throughout the year. Another way your pharmacy works for your health and financial stability.

Building a positive relationship with your pharmacist is one of the most important relationships you will have in your medical family but like with the other members of your medical family if you don't get the customer service you feel you deserve find another pharmacy immediately. There are more options for pharmacies than doctors, so no excuses allowed!

That's the beauty of your medical family as opposed to your real family. You had no say in your real family members, other than your spouse, but you have the ability to pick, choose and keep every member of your medical family, so choose wisely. Your medical family from your doctor to your pharmacist will help shape your quality of life from a health and financial standpoint. Take it upon yourself to ensure those relationships are built on trust, honesty and open communications, which enables or produces mutual respect. It's your life so take responsibility to ensure you get the most out of it, especially within your medical family.

...8...

Your dental and pharmaceutical needs are of extreme importance to your overall health. Don't underestimate either!

9

Caregivers…One Of The Hardest Jobs On Earth

Aside from being a parent, being a caregiver could go down as the hardest job on earth, especially if the patient is a loved one. Caregivers, without a doubt, rate as one of the most important and influential resources in not only the patient's life, but the quality of life for the entire family as well. For those of us who are so blessed to have a primary caregiver that's by our side through thick and thin, happy and sad, good and bad, richer and broke, pleasant and attitude, cooperative and stubborn, understanding and confusion, and night and day, we are the luckiest people on earth. If you don't recognize how much better off you are, regardless of how you feel healthwise, you better start recognizing!

There are many types of primary caregivers. In certain situations it might be a parent, son or daughter that provides the everyday care a patient needs in order to survive. Other situations arise where a grand-child must step in and take care of his/her elderly grandparent or adult children take care of an elderly parent, which can bring on different needs than taking care of someone who is chronically ill. If you have no family, you might turn to a special friend or neighbor, but the reality is those situations are rare because the responsibility of being a primary caregiver is tremendous and alters the caregiver's personal life. If you're in a situation dependant on a friend or neighbor on a regular/daily basis, please understand how special that person is. Then there are the caregivers by occupation. Although they might get paid for their ser-vices, it doesn't change the fact of how important they are to a patient's quality of life and how special they are for choosing that occupation, so be just as thankful for them as well.

For the sake of this book when I refer to the primary caregiver, because it's what I have personal experience with as a patient, I'm re-ferring primarily to your spouse or the person who lives with you. My definition of spouse is the person with whom you're either married or live with and have a personal, probably romantic, relationship with on a daily basis. Your spouse could be your husband or wife, live in boyfriend or girlfriend, or live in partner. The makeup of the relationship doesn't matter, except maybe to those who have nothing better to do in their own lives than worry about how others live. What matters is that person is emotionally attached and dedicated to the well being of their spouse. I understand this situation all too well because my wife has been by my side from the day we met and I understand how difficult I can be.

In order to build a successful patient/caregiver relationship the basic concepts of honesty, trust and open communications, leading to mutual respect, plus remembering a relationship is a two way street, holds just as true as it does with any relationship. Just because someone has a chronic health condition and might need assistance at times doesn't mean he/she doesn't need positive relationships in their lives as well. In fact we may need positive support even more because there are many times when we feel useless and all alone. Because of the uniqueness of a patient/caregiver relationship, especially from a spouse standpoint, there are additional emotions that apply.

One of the toughest emotions a caregiver to a loved one experiences is the emotion of helplessness. When you're the patient, although you might be in a lot of pain or depression, you at least understand what's going on with your health, but as a caregiver all you can do is imagine. Regardless of the situation, be it health or some other moment in life, unless you're the one experiencing the situation firsthand you really don't know what a person is experiencing physically, or even more so, mentally and emotionally. Not truly knowing how a loved one feels can cause a feeling of helplessness that can be extremely difficult to deal with from a mental and emotional aspect. Even more so when the patient is your spouse, parent, child or another close family member.

Having to sit back and watch as your loved one is given treatments or is experiencing pain yet there's nothing you can do to ease the pain, can drive a person crazy with helplessness. We all want to help those we love and most of us would actually trade places with them in a heartbeat if we could, but we can't. All we can do is try and do all we can to ensure our loved ones are as comfortable as possible. The helpless feeling of not being able to make it all better is an emotion caregivers must learn to deal with on a regular basis.

To add to this emotion is the fact all patients are unique individuals therefore every person has unique ways of handling life's situations, especially their own health needs. As a caregiver you want the patient to do as you would do, but that's just not reality. It can be extremely frustrating for a caregiver to feel if only they would do "this", instead of "that", because "this" is how you would deal with it. The thing is for this individual "that" works better for them. As a caregiver you can, and should, give your opinion regarding how you feel are ways that would benefit the patient and make their life easier or less painful but you can only give advice, not make your way the only way. Your way might be great for you but a disaster for someone else.

Grieving is a perfect example of the point I'm trying to make here. The cause for people to grieve is always the same for everyone…someone close to you died. However how an individual grieves is unique to everyone. Some individuals need to have people around them while others want to be alone. Some individuals want to talk about their emotions and reminisce about old times while others just want to meditate with their thoughts and emotions. Some individuals need to get right back to work or to their normal routines while others need time away from the daily grind or maybe never return to a specific routine. Some individuals are very emotional while others might take years to even shed a tear. Some individuals seek counseling while others seek peace from religious readings. Whose way is right or wrong? The answer is simple, but yet complicated. They're all right. It's an individual's unique makeup that determines the best way for them to grieve just like it's an individual's unique makeup that determines the best way for him/her to deal with their health situation.

Be it grieving or health, as a loved one or caregiver, you want to ease the pain an individual experiences by having them act as you would act because, as a human being, we all feel how we deal with obstacles is the best way for everyone. That's just human nature. It's also wrong! As a caregiver the first thing you must do is figure out, understand and accept the best way your patient deals with their health situation. Don't try and force your philosophy on someone else. Make suggestions, yes, but don't force because that will only drive the patient away and thus cause more damage than good. Each individual has a unique personality and just because they become ill doesn't change that fact. We don't all become programmed robots when we endure chronic health conditions or old age. As a caregiver you're not the programmer but instead the supporter. Never forget to treat us as the individuals we are, not as a computer program.

Let's take this logic one step further because I don't want you to confuse allowing us to be individuals and to deal with our health situations in our own way with doing what you have to do as a caregiver to ensure we, as patients, stay as healthy as we can. When it comes down to it, our caregiver is our lifeline and there are going to be times when, as a caregiver, you're going to have to do things that might be uncomfortable for everyone, but necessary such as we have discussed when it comes to addressing body odor or bad breath.

When you're sick there are many times when you'll be out of it and not even realize it. I've had many experiences where I thought I was doing fine but later found things such as financial paperwork or the way I interacted with other people was out of the norm and obvious to everyone, except me. I remember one time at a local neighborhood market I had a lady who I interacted with on a casual basis tell me it was so good to see me smile again. I knew I had been having a rough time the past month or so but didn't realize it was that obvious to people I only encountered every now and then for small talk.

Another example was while my father was in home hospice and his health was declining. My mother had to figure out when it was time to take over certain tasks because, regardless of what my father thought he was doing or what had worked in the past, the reality was he wasn't doing the task correctly as a result of his declining health. A couple of examples were doing the financial books and driving. These were hard decisions for her to make and enforce, but, even more so, it was hard on my father from a mental and emotional standpoint, because he had to admit he was not capable from a health standpoint to function in this manner anymore. Although he accepted his fate and the inevitable changes to his life with dignity, it still had to be a hard fact to admit to himself. He was a strong man to accept an inevitable fate the way he did. It's times like this when our caregivers must look at the reality of the situation, step in and let us know something is wrong or some action needs to take place in a tactful but yet forceful manner.

This can and will be difficult for the caregiver because if we don't realize we're slipping then we sure don't want to hear about it. Our reaction will probably be negative towards you, but, so be it, we need to hear it before we get worse. Common situations include when the patient isn't taking his/her medications as he/she should. If we ignore your suggestions it might be necessary to inform our doctor…with us present. Yes, call us out!

I had a friend and fellow sarcoidosis patient in New York whose wife would call him out during doctor's appointments and it would always lead to a spirited confrontation outside the office. It even got to the point he didn't want her to go with him but regardless she was always by his side. However, at the end of the day he knew how blessed he was to have someone who loved him so much she would put herself in a situation that made him mad and caused him to vent on her because she knew it was best for his health. It would have been easier to just ignore the wrongs and keep peace but that's not what loved ones are supposed to do and definitely not what caregivers are supposed to do. One of the last things he told me was how blessed he was to have this special woman for a wife.

It's a fine line between allowing a person to do what's best for them and understanding what the caregiver is doing is only causing the patient harm. This is another situation where mutual respect comes into play. Without respect you aren't going to listen to a person anyway and if you know you can do whatever you want and your caregiver isn't going to stand up to you then I doubt if you had respect in that relationship from the start.

As a caregiver you have to develop thick skin because a sick person will probably either attack you verbally or ignore you when confronted which can be very frustrating to the point of making you mad or bitter. Although no one should endure abuse, and that's not what I'm suggesting, just be tolerant. Side effects from medications, hormone changes, tiredness, frustration, feelings of uselessness, resentment, guilt and many other factors cause us not to be ourselves. Again, I'm not justifying our inappropriate actions, just explaining them. As a caregiver, understand the difference and step up when we need you. After all you're our lifelines and no one ever said being a caregiver was easy!

Resentment is another emotion that can come into the patient/caregiver relationship. Resentment can be a damaging emotion to an individual and the relationship. Resentment can come from several angles. As a chronically ill patient you could be in a situation where you're unable to work. This can affect both parties negatively if you let it. As the patient you might feel out of control of your own life, especially if you've been the primary financial provider all of your life. Now you're in a situation where your spouse is responsibly for going to work for not only the money, but more importantly, to ensure the family has health care benefits as well. As time passes this can wear on an individual and all of a sudden without warning resentment sets in. Next thing you know you're taking innocent comments personally and reacting as such. You start to feel useless and fall into a state of depression resulting in your health getting worse and thus the quality of life for the entire family suffers, not to mention your relationship.

On the flip side as the caregiver or provider now you find yourself going to work while your spouse stays home. You understand the reasons why he/she can't work but sometimes you just have one of those days at work and it just pisses you off you're the only one working. At home you find every little thing you can to nag about and make comments that hit below the belt on a regular basis. You constantly complain you're the only one working and give examples of other people "like your loved one" who do this or that, even though "their" situation really is nothing like that of your loved one. Deep down you know it, but venting sure makes you feel better. As time goes on you forget how bad things were for your spouse when he/she was working or how serious his/her health situation really is because resentment has made you forget …until something happens and it's too late!

As we know, relationships are hard enough for any two people to build and maintain but relationships between people where one is healthy and the other lives with a chronic health condition can be even more difficult. You both must be aware and do all you can not to let those helpless feelings, frustration or resentment take over and destroy what you have built. Understand things change in life and just because a person can do something today doesn't mean he/she can do those things tomorrow. I think this is the number one complaint I hear from patients, especially sarcoidosis patients since a lot of us "don't look sick". The healthy members will become unhappy and frustrated because the chronically ill members can't do something they used to be able to do with them even though they look like they can from the outside looking in. As a result, instead of finding something else to do together, they end up terminating the relationship.

I think one advantage I have in my relationship with my wife, although things have still changed during our relationship and we're still both human, is the fact when she met me I was already in bad shape in regard to sarcoidosis and had quit doing most of the things I used to do, such as play basketball regularly. As a result she doesn't have anything to compare me to from a healthy/sick perspective, only progressive changes that occur over time in our relationship. Although I wish we could have enjoyed life when I was full of energy, in reality this fact has probably strengthened our relationship and kept out a level of resentment.

I understand you might have started your life together with many dreams and one of you becoming chronically ill was not in the plans, but no one knows what tomorrow brings. Personally speaking I think, although it's a tough situation, anyone who leaves their spouse because they have become ill didn't unconditionally love their spouse or was not committed to the relationship to begin with. Regardless of your logic behind why you can't handle it anymore or feel you don't deserve to live your life in this manner, you're weak and wrong! If you get upset with my statement or tell me your spouse told you to leave because it was unfair to you, then I'll give you my, and only my, opinion once again…you're weak and wrong. You should have thought about that "before" you committed to the relationship! Remember in life "what goes around – comes around". Just pray you're never in need of a caregiver or loved one.

I tell my wife she will never have to worry about anyone taking care of her if she is ever in need. During the time I've known her she has taken care of me unconditionally, was the primary caregiver for her grandmother for years, took care of her mother in her time of need until her death, gives her daughter unconditionally support, along with our granddaughter, and shows compassion for those close to her. As a result God will ensure there's someone available to take care of her because of her caring actions. It might be her daughter, granddaughter, a friend, or me, but someone will be there. You never know when it will be your time to need assistance so please keep that reality in mind before you abandon your loved one in need or put your own agenda ahead of caring for a loved one.

Not only are there mental and emotional challenges, there are physical challenges as well. We've discussed several already and I want to touch on an important responsibility we touched on briefly and that's the responsibility of knowing where all of the required information is located for the patient and being up to date on the status of the patient's health situation, including medications and documented on their HIPAA sheet. This is a responsibility that could be the difference between life and death!

One thing I stress that all patients should do is to wear some type of medical alert identification either by necklace or bracelet. In addition it's even more important to keep a card or letter (other than your personal notebook you use for your doctors) in your wallet or purse at all times detailing your medical condition and noted on your medical alert jewelry. I also keep one in both glove compartments of both our cars and in my luggage when I travel. The information should include the details of your medical condition, current medications, dosages, insurance information, doctor contacts and emergency contacts. With updated technology the use of USB or extended storage devices are starting to be used as well. These devices can be on a necklace, a key ring, or in your pocket or purse. You can store your medical information on them, then they can be inserted into any USB port on a computer or laptop and your information retrieved. In times of emergency the easier this information is available, and more detailed, the better your chances for success is increased. In cases such as mine the lack of this information could be deadly!

Sometimes having your information on you might not be enough. In times of emergency when chaos can runs wild, even the most well trained professionals, might overlook medical alerts or not check your personal items for documentation. It's not so much their fault, although they're trained to look for such information on a patient, as it is human nature and the moment, but reality is what it is. It can be critical that the caregiver not only knows where the information is located but also will be aggressive enough to ensure the information gets into the right hands. In emergency situations a caregiver must make sure he/she is on top of the situation while still allowing the medical personnel to do their jobs.

Another reality is in emergency room situations where detailed medical records are not readily available, although some medical facilities are developing extensive online medical record access for their patients. But who can ensure when your emergency arises you will be at a facility with detailed online access? In cases such as mine, where a number of medical professionals don't have an in depth familiarity with sarcoidosis and the life or death effect sarcoidosis has on what might seem like an insignificant symptom such as vomiting, sometimes special instructions need to be relayed via the caregiver. My wife knows what needs to happen at times like this more so than some of the medical professionals treating me. This isn't a knock on the medical professionals or saying she knows their jobs better than they do, a lot of them simply won't listen to the patient, if the patient is able to communicate, or to the caregiver, which can be deadly. She knows the direction that needs to be followed and more importantly who needs to be contacted or else I'm in deadly trouble as a result of a seemingly insignificant symptom.

No one can know everything and some conditions, such as sarcoidosis, aren't detailed as much as others in medical training, plus my detailed medical chart, aside from my detailed information I provide, is not readily available the majority of the time. Being able to convey this information to the appropriate medical professionals when they are not listening may at times take required/tactful aggressive action and stubbornness in order to get them to do what is needed. Let me give you an example about what I mean.

It was the end of March 2005 and about 2:00 A.M. I woke up feeling funny. I went to the bathroom and spent the next 15 minutes or so having a serious case of diarrhea. I returned to bed and about 45 minutes later my wife and I commented on the still lingering strong smell of my bowel movements. I've never smelled anything like that odor! Even though both of us sleep with a CPAP mask the smell was as strong as it was 45 minutes prior. Around 3:15 A.M., still feeling weird I tried to make it to the bathroom once again but this time I started to experience serious problems.

At first I started experiencing difficulty breathing, as it was hard to catch my breath. In addition I felt a tingling all over my body, especially in my head. I was very cold but yet sweating heavily. The left side of my body was getting numb and I couldn't stop yawning. The next thing I knew I was gagging for air and trying to vomit but couldn't. After a little mucus came up, I vomited a couple of times, including some blood, while still continuing to gag, cough and gasp for air as my chest was pounding like nothing I had experienced before. Slowly I fell into a state of semi-unconsciousness.

When situations such as these arise it can be a life threatening experience for me because of the abnormal nature of my immune system caused by pituitary sarcoidosis, although I had never quite experienced all of these symptoms at once. When I vomit uncontrollably I need to be injected with steroids in order to get my immune system to react properly. Otherwise my blood pressure will drop resulting in me suffering a stroke or even death. So it's a serious situation, although to some it might just seem like someone is "just" throwing up.

I remember my wife telling me she had called 911 as I sunk slowly to the floor. The next thing I remember was an EMS technician was over me asking if I could hear him. I responded, "Yes", as they slowly helped me to a chair as I was still gasping for air. In the meantime my wife had provided them with my medical information and medications along with my insurance information. As they asked me questions she was also answering questions for me, when I was unable to communicate; although I could hear them asking me the question there were times I couldn't speak. Based on how I was feeling and reacting, along with my medical history, they decided without hesitation to rush me to the emergency room about 10 minutes away. I must say I've always had a positive experience when dealing with any and all EMS technicians, personally and with my mother-in-law, in both the cities of Detroit and Southfield, Michigan. My hat goes off to you all!

A side note…if you hear an EMS vehicle approaching please stop and pull your vehicle all the way to the right side of the road and don't just stop where you are. My wife rode with the EMS vehicle when they took her mother to the emergency room and it's amazing what the EMS drivers have to put up with from inconsiderate drivers. Next time you hear an EMS vehicle ask yourself, "What would I want other drivers to do if one of my loved ones or myself were in the vehicle in an extreme emergency situation?" Without even knowing your actions could be affecting the outcome of someone's life! Think about that, now back to my story.

I was placed on a stretcher and taken to the ambulance. It was cold outside and I remember how warm it finally was when I was inside the ambulance, as I was already shaking uncontrollably. They called ahead to the emergency room while I was given an IV. When I arrived at the emergency room I was taken directly to a room. Although my endocrinologist has always told me to inform the emergency room of my condition, give them his card for them to contact immediately and for the emergency room staff to give me the priority of a heart attack victim, this was the first time they actually took me directly to a room. Usually in urban emergency rooms you're made to wait for a long time or if you're taken back it is to meet the time guarantee a lot of emergency rooms advertise in the urban medical facilities to get your business these days, or you're still put on a stretcher in the hallway for quite a while or must wait for treatment. Maybe because this time my heart was actually a problem it made a difference.

Either way while in the room the nurses and doctors who were examining me still didn't seem to take my condition as serious as it was, but instead took it more so of a person with an irregular fast heartbeat who was vomiting. My wife arrived and began telling them of my condition in detail and the fact I needed the IV with the steroids as soon as possible. In fact she was the one holding the bucket as I continued to vomit while the others in the room kind of stood around and watched, although I must assume/hope they were actually doing something, as my mind frame was not the best at the time. She kept telling the doctor treating me to call my endocrinologist and he would tell him what to do but they didn't seem to believe her. The doctor just told her, in a snobby way, he needed to check my vitals because the endocrinologist (who is very respected at this medical center) would just ask him those questions. My wife kept on more aggressively telling him that was wrong and time was our enemy! "If you just tell him it's Gil Barr he will tell you immediately what to do! The longer you wait the worse he will become! We've been dealing with this for years!" my wife told him directly and confidently. But he and the nurses just looked at her as if what she was saying was going in one ear and out the other. "What does she know? We're the medical professionals here! Sounds to us like she's talking by way of emotion!" was the attitude being displayed while my condition got worse and started to enter the danger zone.

Finally she just walked out (it was about 5:00 A.M. by now) and called my endocrinologist directly from her cell phone and left a detailed message describing what was going on. A few minutes after she returned to the room the same doctor who didn't want to call him came in and said my endocrinologist had called and wanted them to give me the IV of steroids my wife had been trying to tell him I needed. Of course he had even more of an attitude in his tone and we didn't see him anymore the rest of our emergency room visit. Who cares! If not for the knowledge of my condition by my wife and her aggressive follow-up when no one would listen to her who knows where I might be now. That's what a caregiver does when it's needed!

This is a problem I've experienced many times over in emergency room situations and with other doctors as well. I remember one doctor wanted to bring interns around to ask me questions because I had diabetes insipidus, as it was rare to see an actual patient in person, instead of calling my endocrinologist for advice regarding my condition, as time for me to safely obtain the IV was ticking away. The examples have piled up over the years, as it seems some doctors don't want to admit they don't know as much about sarcoidosis and the effect it has on me. Everyone understands you can't know everything and sarcoidosis is still mysterious, and again not taught as it should be in medical training, but when you won't admit to not knowing as a doctor, you put our lives at stake.

I know I sound like a broken record regarding this subject, but if so it's because I've been in this situation so much it seems like I'm spinning on the turntable uncontrollably with the Dee Jay on break. Some of you may take it as me being bitter and negative as well but like I told you in the introduction you have to face bad situations from a reality standpoint in order to eliminate the negative from occurring again. This is one of those situations. The bottom line is this attitude by some (and I want to stress "some") medical staff professionals is not only unacceptable, but also dangerous for us all! I plead with any medical professional reading this now never to be afraid of admitting you might need help or don't fully understand, but instead always be afraid of the consequences of not admitting your lack of knowledge by being aware of the results of your failure to seek help might have on your patient and family. It happens more often than the medical community wants to admit.

Eventually I was admitted to the hospital to monitor my heartbeat and in a couple of days my heartbeat was back to normal, at least for me, and I was released. My endocrinologist thought I had a slight heart attack based on my symptoms. We didn't spend too much time worrying about why but instead concentrated on getting me back to myself and how to prevent this from happening again. I did learn later on I was doing the right thing by coughing and taking deep breaths, as this is what you should do if you are alone and having a heart attack. For me, this time around, everything turned out okay except for a month or so my wife became overprotective. It's the reality check a longtime caregiver gets when things happen.

My caregiver having the knowledge of my health information was a lifesaver for me, on more than one occasion, and it's critical all caregivers are aware of how to find and relay the vital information to the right people or take it upon themselves to ensure the right people are contacted, when needed. Preparation is the key so if you must review from time to time what you have to do, do it! When the time comes, there isn't room for error. Instead of a fire drill, conduct a health drill. When it becomes the real deal too much is at stake. Remember there are no dress rehearsals in emergency situations!

To top it off a personal benefit my wife received by knowing she did all she could was it didn't allow the most costly emotion to a patient/caregiver relationship or individual's mental outlook sneak into her mental makeup…GUILT.

…9…

Sometimes life puts us in situations for a reason and the fact you find yourself a caregiver is one of those situations. God never gives you too much responsibility. Although a caregiver is not easy by any stretch of the imagination, upholding your responsibility to the best of your ability will provide you with eternal rewards!

10
Guilt

Guilt is one of the most powerful emotions an individual can experience and a high percentage of the time, especially in health related relationships, is the root to the tree of negativity. From the time we were children learning life guilt has been a part of our life. Whether you accidentally broke a friend's toy or maybe accidentally hurt someone while playing, guilt was something you had to learn to handle. As a teenager if you followed the wrong crowd and made fun of the un-cool kid or said something cruel to your parents, afterwards guilt hopefully took over your mind and made you feel miserable, causing you to learn how to make amends. If you were mischievous and took something that wasn't yours or destroyed someone's property for no reason, I pray guilt made you want to correct your wrong as well. Some people live with guilt for life as a result of how they treated a person or maybe because of something they never got around to doing or saying to them before it was too late. Guilt can tear your heart out and make you question your own morals. We must all learn how to avoid feeling guilty by our actions and when we as human beings do what human beings sometimes do, causing guilt to enter our lives, we must learn how to deal with it and learn from it. Guilt serves no positive purpose and must be dealt with head on, especially when it involves patient/caregiver relationships.

Guilt sets in for several reasons. As a patient needing support from a loved one you, at times, start to feel like you're depriving your loved one of life as they should live it because so much time and effort is spent caring for you. Even if you're independent not being able to do the things you used to do, causes guilt to set in. A common scenario is once again a patient not being able to work a "regular" job due to his/her health. For most of us, especially those of us who have worked all our lives and been the primary financial provider for our family and ourselves, this can be something that constantly weighs heavily on our minds. Even if everyone in the family understands why you're on disability and actually encouraged you to stop working because of the reality of your health, plus you still bring in money on a monthly basis that contributes to the family, the scenario still causes guilt to build up and over time can cause problems within the relationship. Watching your loved one get up and go to work on a daily basis, especially on days you feel good, causes you to feel guilty or useless. This is a normal feeling for anyone committed to a relationship. So how do you deal with it?

For one, as the patient, do everything you can physically and emotionally to pull your weight in the relationship which will make you feel good about yourself. Everyone wants to feel useful! There are no set rules for a man or woman and there are a lot of areas in a relationship that needs to be covered. Determine what you can do from a physical standpoint and do it. I know this can be tough, especially when you're alone and not feeling good, because I experience it myself. My wife works a "regular" job while I stay home. Even though I write and have work relating to my books or supporting other patients that takes up a lot of my day, I still don't have the responsibility to be some place for a certain amount of time every workday. However there are certain routines and responsibilities I maintain, when physically able, that contribute to our family and keeps guilt from entering my emotional being…most days that is.

I get up, see my wife off to work, take my medications, eat, shower and get dressed. This is important because it gives me a sense of going to work or doing something other than sitting around in my pajamas feeling like I'm lounging. As simple as that routine may sound, it changes my complete frame of mind in a positive manner. Next I go to my "office" (in the basement), balance the books to ensure no one has stolen our identity, answer any e-mails or phone calls, then write for a few hours until around 11:00 or 11:30 when my stomach says it's time for lunch. I'll fix some lunch or go out (one of my weaknesses is I love to eat out anytime of the day), then do my daily walk for at least 30 minutes along with running any errands or chores that need to be done. Depending on what needed to be done I'll either go back to my office or start preparing dinner around 3:30 or so, depending on what I'm cooking. After dinner I'll spend quality time with my wife until around 8:00 PM when we go to our separate televisions for our different taste's in what we watch. Around 10:00 or 11:00 PM I'll go to bed.

That's a "regular" routine day for me. Of course there are days when my health doesn't allow me to do what I normally do and on those days I just do what I have to do to make it to the next day where I'll hopefully be able to get back to "normal".

My responsibilities around the house, that I can physically do, include doing the laundry, keeping and balancing the financial books, ensuring all of the bills are paid, doing the grocery and household shopping, running any household or personal errands (mine or my wife's) that need to be done, making sure dinner is prepared, and most importantly, spend quality time with my wife and allow her to vent about her day at work when she gets home. That routine allows me to contribute to the household and at the same time allows me to feel useful.

Now you might ask, and this question can be a source of guilt within a chronically ill patient even if they understand their own feelings, "If you can do all that why can't you get out and work a "regular" job?" I can't answer for you, but in my case it's because my primary reason for not being able to do something on a regular basis, other than when I'm experiencing serious health problems, is chronic fatigue. Take doing the laundry for example. I can put a load of clothes in the washing machine. Later on I put them in the dryer; then when I feel up to it, fold them, which might even be the next day. In other words I'm able to do these responsibilities at my own pace and if for some health reason I can't do them this day, there is always tomorrow. I don't negatively impact a business or let others depending on me down as I did when I couldn't make it into the office for two weeks straight from 1991 to 2002 while at EDS. In the work place you're expected, and have others depending on you as well, to perform everyday at your required time, not when you're able. That's the difference. However even understanding this fact of my life and accepting my reality, guilt can still creep in from time to time.

In these types of situations it's extremely important the caregiver doesn't make comments that open the door for guilt. Although they might just be venting after a bad day, those words, however unintentional, causes guilt to take advantage of an opportunity to make itself at home. "How would you know, all you do is stay home all day?" or "Other people worse off than you can work!" or better yet, and with sarcastic attitude, "If you want to do something, I see you don't have a problem doing that!" are just some examples of statements with rolling eyes and neck circling to go along with them, which might have been said out of frustration caused by something other than their loved one, they simply feel comfortable venting on their loved one. Such statements can cut deep into someone who might already feel subconsciously guilty about their inability to contribute as they used to. After the comments are made the caregiver probably doesn't give what was said a second thought, after all they've vented now and feel better, but I promise you the chronically ill patient hears it over and over in their heads! "Those" looks, outside of your venting, can be just as damaging. You know the ones where the eyes roll up in your head when something is said or maybe when something on television comes on about something sensitive to the chronically ill patient and you give "that" nod of agreement. There's also your lack of interest in the chronically ill patient's day as if to say what they do is not important. Sometimes a lack of words can do more harm than venting.

The best way to minimize guilt from this situation is, like a broken record, honest communications and understanding between the patient and caregiver, on good and bad days. Learn when to give space and when to give comfort. Relationships are mutual so it's extremely critical both parties understand and accept the fate your relationship is in, therefore, allowing you both to vent when necessary but yet still keep the fence sturdy to block guilt from entering the relationship from any angle, as much as possible. When the fence weakens talk about how you feel, and most of all, listen to what your partner is saying. Listening can be more important than venting, for both parties. If I've said it once I've said it a million times, no one can understand how another person feels unless you communicate honestly, regardless of the situation, so listen with an open mind.

Another negative emotion guilt triggers, especially in this type of situation, as we touched on earlier, is more resentment. Caregivers could build resentment towards the chronically ill patient because they feel they're doing everything. Not only do they have to get up for work while the other person might still be in bed, but they also have to fulfill other obligations as well. When they want to do something the chronically ill patient always feels bad or can't make it. They start thinking negative thoughts, they know deep down are wrong, but reality doesn't stop them from thinking negatively anyway because the guilt of your responsibilities and lack of honest communications has caused you to develop resentment. They resent the fact it's always them that seems to be doing the hard tasks for the family and, at this time of their thought process, their spouse or the patient does nothing. I promise you one thing, I know of no patient with chronic health conditions, myself included, who wouldn't in a heartbeat take on the hardest job in the world if the chronic health conditions would disappear…even for one day!

Like relationships, resentment works both ways! As the chronically ill patient you start resenting the fact you feel no one understands how you feel and the struggles you experience just doing the little things in life. "How do they know how I feel? Do they think I enjoy letting people down because of my health? I wish they could live one day in my shoes, that would show them!" are thoughts you experience as self-pity and resentment take over your thought process. "Why me?" makes you resent others in your life who might achieve something you would give anything to be able to do again, regardless of how simple the achievement might have been.

So how do you prevent resentment from destroying your relationship? You know it, honest communications with your loved one and more importantly yourself. You can't feel guilty about having resentment based on your situation. We all feel these emotions during our life. Feeling them is not the problem! Not dealing with them head on and honestly is the issue and what damages the relationship! In a patient/caregiver relationship there's so much at stake other than your feelings. If you're in this type of committed relationship you should already understand this fact of life. Your loved one needs you and you need your loved one so don't allow guilt to build resentment and destroy your relationship of choice. Never forget, your spouse and this relationship was your choice! It might not have started out like this but still it was, and is, your choice.

As a primary caregiver there are other situations, out of your control, that cause your life to change and can be a primary source of guilt, such as feeling obligated to take care of a family member because no one else in the family will step up. Personally I have a philosophy about the responsibilities an individual has in regard to taking care of family members and it goes like this. First everyone has the unconditional obligation to take care of his/her spouse. That's the one family member you picked for your life partner therefore, unless you get a divorce, your spouse is your number one obligation. Second come your children and parents. You brought your children into this world therefore it's your unconditional obligation to take care of them until adulthood. However, your children are always your children and the responsibility to care for them in their time of need is always yours, regardless of how old they are at the time. Granted some children need tough love (with love being the keyword) and as a parent you must decide when those times arise. But the fact remains your children are a product of your upbringing so look very closely at yourself before you ever turn your back on the very individuals you created! In addition you owe your parents unconditional support in their times of need as well. "You start out life depending on your parents and you end life depending on your children." What goes around comes around and just as your parents took care of you in your time of need you owe them the same. Worth noting…because you made a child doesn't make you a parent. My daughter doesn't have my DNA but I see myself in her actions everyday and she is without a doubt my daughter! Each person must look at his/her own unique situation. The bottom line is for those people you consider a parent the unconditional obligation is there for you to care for them when their time of need comes, as they did for you.

Grandchildren and grandparents can also be a responsibility, if the parents or children are not available for whatever reason to care for them properly. Those two groups do fit into my view of obligation but not necessarily unconditional. As mentioned in the previous paragraph, it's the children and parents initial responsibility but like having a spouse on disability, sometimes life gives us a fate out of our control and we must step up. Brothers and sisters fit into this category as well, it's just hard for me to relate to them because I'm an only child.

As far as those other family members such as aunts, uncles, cousins, nephews or nieces, well those are determined on an individual basis. I have some cousins I wouldn't know if I was in line with them at the supermarket and have friends who I owe more to than them for they are truly my brothers. So don't let a distant family member or a family member who only comes to you when they want something, lay a guilt trip on you just because you have the same blood. Yes, blood is thicker than water but unknown or disloyal blood is not thicker than close friendship. Based on my personal philosophy and for the sake of this book, I'm just going to address parents and children.

A very high number of individuals must at some point in their lives make tough decisions regarding the care of their parents. The care could consist of your parents still living independently and your checking on them and assisting them on a daily basis. There are those situations in which your parents come to live with you and your family, putting you in the middle between raising your family and caring for your elderly or disabled parents, which is now being referred to as the "Sandwich Generation" since it happens quite often in today's society. The emotional burden along with the physical stress of either situation can and will be very demanding. You must look closely at your situation and not allow guilt to determine your course of action but instead make logically decisions. Your decisions will affect not only you but also your parents and other family members.

I know none of us want to put our parents in some type of elderly or nursing home if we can help it. However sometimes that's the logical decision when based on the medical needs of the patient not on the caregiver's desire to go on a vacation or some other self-centered motive. Of course finances play a major part in that decision, but barring any financial issues, if you aren't able physically or emotionally to handle the responsibility of caring for your parents you might need to consider other options. Base your decision on what's best for your parents and don't allow guilt or self-indulgence to make the decision for you. No one but your Maker can judge your decision so who cares what others think? Your only concern should be the care of your parents and what's best for them. Making the right decision will mean looking deep into your own life. Don't let guilt cloud your vision!

You must never put yourself or your wants ahead of the responsibility of caring for your parents; they didn't when you needed care. Neglecting your parents in need because of laziness or feeling you have other things better to do is another of guilt's primary accomplice. Not ensuring your parents have enough of the foods they prefer or other little things they enjoy is wrong on your part. The thing is you might only have one opportunity to take care of your loved one therefore you better think of them and not yourself. If not, guilt will be your new life partner. Everyone gets over the grieving process but guilt never truly leaves one's heart. Your parents, wishes or, at the least to the best of your knowledge, should always, when possible, be honored.

Caring for your children is already a huge responsibility. Being a parent is the hardest job in the world…bar none! A parent is the ultimate caregiver. Parenting is a full-time job with consequences resulting from each decision, action and non-action made. There are no manuals to teach you how to be a good parent. Parenting is something you must learn on your own with each child and situation being different. Don't let guilt determine your course of actions. Just because you might have made a mistake the first time doesn't mean you can't learn from it and correct it. You're not your children's friend, you're their parent, so don't let guilt or the fear they might be mad at you keep you from doing what you know is best for them. You set the foundation for the rest of their lives; therefore don't allow guilt to weaken the foundation.

Here are my three rules to being a successful parent. First think of everything your parents did for you that was productive and make sure you do the same. Secondly, think of everything your parents did for you that caused you harm and absolutely had a negative effect on your actions and life; then make sure you don't do the same. Last, think of everything, honestly with the advantage of hindsight, you feel your parents should have done for you, whether you would have liked it or not, that would have had a positive impact on your life and make sure you do those things for your children. Of course when your children become parents themselves they can use the same fundamental rules but since all children are different the actual course of actions will be different as well. Still if you keep these three logical rules as your premise you and your children will be okay.

As with anything else in life there are times when fate just doesn't seem to give you a break. Some might look at the responsibility of raising a child with a chronic health condition or disability as one of those situations. Don't because that child still needs all of the care, guidance and love any other child needs, and then some. In return they can provide the same joy and blessings any non-disabled child will bring into a parent's life. Sometimes even more as you appreciate the little things in life that others take for granted.

In order to provide those needs you as a parent cannot under any circumstance allow guilt or resentment to take over your mental state of mind. It's a normal response to somehow feel the child's condition is your fault, but it's not. It's nobody's fault; therefore don't dwell on it. Obviously this is easier said than done. You must not under any circumstance allow guilt to overcome your responsibility of caring for your child or resentment to cause you to lash out. Special needs takes a special parent and we all have it in us. It might just take a little soul searching to bring it out. Don't be afraid to be yourself or ask for help. You'll do just fine!

Speaking of being yourself, that's one of the most important things about being a successful caregiver and a fact, we as chronically ill patients, regardless of the situation, must remember. How can you take care of us if you don't take care of yourself? Guilt will do all it can to ensure you neglect your own needs and that's something neither you nor the patient can allow.

As a chronically ill patient we all feel guilty from time to time for needing assistance and taking away from what we see as a normal life for you. In the same tone, we can't allow guilt to fail to give you a break from us when the situation arises. Giving our caregivers a guilt-free break is the ultimate gift of love and understanding a chronically ill patient can give a caregiver. We must allow our caregiver to get away from us, if just for a night out, and let him/her get away without feeling the guilt of leaving us. In most situations we can make preparations to ensure a little away time can be achieved. It's not only something we should do; it's something we must do…for our own good.

I don't know about you but I would give anything to be able to spend one day without having to deal with my health situation. Just to be able to wake up refreshed, not take any medications, be able to do whatever I wanted without pain or worry, eat what I wanted, take no insulin, play basketball and go to sleep without pain or wearing a CPAP mask…just one day! I know that will never be a reality for me, but I can make sure my wife has time away from me where she doesn't have to deal directly with my health. It might only be a night out with the girls or maybe a weekend trip. One thing I might do is go to Florida and visit my family while she stays at home in Detroit, away from my health issues. Sure she'll still think about me and probably worry a little as well, but at least she doesn't have to deal with the physical and mental aspects of my illness firsthand. That in itself is a well deserved break.

When giving this wonderful break to your caregiver and to ensuring it works you must remember it's guilt-free. Don't make innocent comments such as, "You have a good time I should be okay." Should be okay? No, you will be okay! Make sure of it. Depending on the break, make sure you have contact numbers and have made arrangements for someone else to help you with things you might not be able to do for yourself. Have food that's already prepared or you can prepare available. Plan some activity for yourself even if it's as simple as having a movie or a sporting event to watch or reading a good book. Not only make sure you're prepared to enjoy the break but more importantly make sure your caregiver truly understands you will be okay and is comfortable with the game plan beforehand thus...GUILT-FREE!

As a caregiver it's just as important you recognize when you need a break and when you can take a break. Don't let guilt cause you to burn yourself out. This will not only cause you harm but will negatively impact your patient and all of the others who need your support. Superman and Wonder Woman are cartoon characters. You're human. Never forget that! There's nothing in this world to feel guilty about when it comes to being burned out. Don't allow guilt, be it from someone else or internally, to force you to harm yourself by being blind to your own needs. Take a guilt-free break for not only yourself, but for your loved ones as well, because they will benefit just as much as you will from your reenergized state of mind. If the guilt-free break is properly prepared for there will be no harm done and only positive results will follow. Depending on the situation it could be a simple afternoon spent alone or shopping. Taking a guilt-free break doesn't mean flying out of the country when your patient needs your attention. Your break needs to be based on the patient's needs. Maybe a few hours away is what you need. Either way, it's okay to worry a little while you're gone or check in to make sure everything's okay; just make sure you're able to free your mind in the time you have away. That's the ultimate objective so everyone benefits.

After you were able to have a successful break, please don't put an

Aunt Bee guilt trip on yourself upon your return. By this I'm referring to an episode on the old Andy Griffith television series where Aunt Bee finally went out of town but when she came back she saw Andy and Opie had managed okay. Actually they had busted their behinds to clean up at the last minute so they would make Aunt Bee proud. Then Andy started to think that because they pretended to manage okay she might feel she wasn't needed, and he was right. When they went to pick Aunt Bee up a neighbor came to the house and cleaned up, causing Aunt Bee to feel as if she wasn't needed. This logic only makes the guilt-free break useless. If you properly prepare beforehand, as a good caregiver will do, then anyone should be able to manage based on the situation. That doesn't mean the caregiver is less needed or the patient is less loved. No, that's guilt destroying a good thing once again. Actually it just shows how much the caregiver is needed and how well he/she takes on his/her responsibilities because, after all, the caregiver is the one who ensured everything would run smoothly.

Just to clarify, when I'm talking about the guilt-free break I'm not referring to those situations when a patient is most likely at the end of their time. Such examples might be a cancer patient or a parent whose age most likely will not let them survive much longer. In those cases you just have to continue support because putting your parent away or taking personal time for your own pleasure might be a guilt partnership in the making, especially if they die while you're gone or planning to go. No, I'm primarily referring to the caregiver who takes care of a chronically ill patient such as myself. If something happened to happen to me while my wife was gone then that was just God's calling and my wife should not feel guilt of any kind. Recognize the difference! Sometimes we have to do what we have to do.

Patient to patient - don't take it personally! Your caregiver needs a break from your health situation because he/she is human. Your self-pity will prevent them from enjoying their break thus not achieving the goal of reenergizing the caregiver in order that he/she can continue to take care of you. If they didn't want to be with you, do you really think they would need a guilt-free break? No, they would already be gone. If you must look at it from a selfish standpoint, ask yourself this. If you need help do you want a physically and mentally worn out person responding or do you want a responsive person capable of handling your situation to come running to your aid? I think the answer is obvious.

However, there's something else you need to consider besides having a physically and mentally drained caregiver, or anyone else in your life for that matter, who is not going to respond in the proper timeframe when you actually need help. You must never cry wolf! I've touched on the crying wolf theory briefly several times so far during this book but when it comes to your caregiver the impact can be even more negative from both a physical and mental perspective. Your caregiver must be able to believe what you tell him/her in regard to your needs. We've already established being a caregiver, especially for a loved one, involves more than just the chronically ill patient but other responsibilities as well. It's a physically and mentally demanding responsibility and the last thing anyone needs is to have unnecessary straws added on to the pile. That's how you get to the last straw and nobody wants to be the victim of a last straw!

As patients we have to understand the world doesn't evolve around only us. It can't! Everyone loves attention, in fact a lot of folks will fake or exaggerate an illness just to get sole attention, causing your caregiver to stop whatever else he/she is doing to react or care for you when the reality is you don't need his/her undivided attention. Why are you adding extra stress, both physically and mentally, by requiring attention when it is not needed? After physically attending to you the unfinished task has to still be completed. Mentally you have now increased his/her concern for your so-called need. Don't you think they have enough stress as it is? If you understand your body, you should know when you're in serious need for help and when you can suck it up. Being sick, especially with chronic health problems, is not an easy life. Believe me I know! That's also why it's called chronic. We must deal with pain, loneliness, depression and feelings of frustration, to name a few, on a daily basis. However that doesn't give us the right to take advantage of our caregivers and that's exactly what you're doing when you cry wolf. As Gomer Pyle would say, "Selfish, selfish, selfish!" Yeah, I used to watch a lot of the Andy Griffith Show as a kid.

The real danger to crying wolf is eventually it will fall on deaf ears and that has dramatic consequences for everyone. People will only continue to react so long, regardless of their love or situation, when each time they react it's a false alarm. I think we have all experienced, at least once, in our lives having someone tell us something is wrong and after dropping everything we might be doing we find out nothing was wrong. Think back to the feelings you had once you realized you had wasted your time and effort and the person knew it all along. Now imagine already being stressed out, on an emotional edge and behind in your responsibilities how you would feel when you realize you have been called once again for a false alarm. Now comes the dangerous part. Imagine how you will feel the next time you're called! I would be willing to bet the first time you were called you dropped everything without hesitation or regard and rushed to the aid of your loved one. However this time, as the straw pile has begun to grow, I bet you finished what you were doing before you went to the aid of your loved one. The problem is, what if this time it was the real deal? The future of both the patient and the caregiver is impacted if the answer is "it was!"

From a patient's standpoint your life could be at stake. In my case when I start vomiting uncontrollably and possibly pass out, if someone doesn't come running and react in a timely manner, I'm in serious trouble. I want to make this clear to whoever is reading this book and to the world, if I cry for help come as fast as you can. As a patient we need our caregivers and support resources, including our doctors, to understand this fact and trust in our word, so don't take advantage of them. It will only come back to hurt you in the end and at that point the only person you can blame is looking at you from the mirror.

You're causing guilt to set in on your loved one as well. Do I go or do I stay? That's a question caregivers should never have to ask themselves and the only reason they would is if the patient has cried wolf in the past. When the patient calls a caregiver should understand the importance and seriousness of the situation by how he/she was called. The only way he/she can understand the urgency of the situation is for the patient to be honest and the caregiver trust in the patient's assessment of the situation, based on past experiences.

The reverse crying wolf theory is just as damaging. This is where the patient never asks for help and downplays his/her health needs as if they will go away on their own or whether the patient feels guilty for needing help. The guilt a loved one feels when the patient has suffered unnecessarily without asking for help can be a lifelong burden, especially after he/she is gone. Why couldn't he/she have asked for my help? Didn't he/she feel comfortable enough with our relationship to let me know how he/she was feeling? Didn't he/she know if he/she had let me know how he/she felt he/she wouldn't be in the situation he/she is in today? These are just some of the guilt related questions a loved one will ask themselves with no possible chance for an answer as now it's too late. As a patient we might think we're doing everyone a favor by keeping things to ourselves or it's too personal for us to involve our loved ones but in the end we only hurt those we love by leaving them with an unnecessary guilt complex.

I understand some of us, I'm one of those people, don't want others feeling sorry for us or we want to stay independent as much as possible. We must understand the difference in being independent, selfish or stupid, because not taking care of yourself or listening to your body signs when you know full well something is wrong and you need help is not right! Don't leave avoidable guilt on your loved ones. As so often the case, the solution is being honest with yourself and your loved ones about how you feel and what you need. No one can help you if he/she doesn't understand what you need and no one will help you if you keep asking for needs that don't exist. As always the responsibility for your own health comes back to you!

Using your health for other emotions is wrong as well and could be deadly. There's nothing wrong with being lonely or wanting a loved one to spend time with you. Communicate honestly how you feel to them. Tell them you would love to have dinner and spend some quality time with them without dealing with your health situation. Sometime as individuals we want affection or to be held by the one we love. Using a health crisis is not the way to achieve companionship.

Your relationship with your caregiver must be open enough where you can express how you honestly feel without guilt. Listening and understanding the feelings and needs of both the patient and caregiver is critical to the success of the relationship and in turn the success of the patient's health. Under no circumstance should guilt be allowed to dictate the response, emotions or feelings of anyone. Learn to understand when guilt has entered the situation; then deal with it as guilt can, will and has destroyed many relationships throughout history. Don't let it destroy yours!

One last thought I want to leave you with regarding the patient/caregiver relationship, along with the parent and friend relationships as well. Everyone likes to hear those two magic words "Thank You!" and everyone wants to feel appreciated. As a caregiver, parent, and friend, especially if you're a good one, you will be taken for granted at some point in the relationship or at least feel like you are. Don't let it bother you. Instead take it as the ultimate compliment it is. The fact of the matter is in order to be taken for granted you have to come through each and every time. Why else would someone take for granted you were going to be there? To be taken for granted, I feel, portrays the fact you're doing it right. Still as a human being we all like to feel appreciated and caregivers, parents, and friends are no different.

So patients of all types remember those two magic words for your caregiver. Remember to say "Thank You" to your friends and children, especially your adult children who take care of you. There are a lot of offspring who find every excuse not to uphold their responsibilities to their parents for selfish reasons. Show acknowledgment of your appreciation by simply saying, "Thank You!" You might not understand it now but those two magical words will make anyone in your life on which you depend so happy. For all those who don't hear any magical words from your patients, children, parents, friends or loved ones, keep on doing what you're doing. Being taken for granted means you're doing it right and without a doubt is the ultimate compliment! So for them I say to you, "THANK YOU!"

…10…

Sometimes you only have one opportunity to care for a loved one. Based on how you react or don't react to your obligation will live inside you throughout eternity!

11
When The Patient Becomes The Caregiver

For the majority of my life with sarcoidosis I looked at caregivers from a patient's perspective. Sure, I had some past indirect experiences such as my daughter being sick and there was nothing I could do about it but try and make her comfortable - but that's really just technically being a parent. There were the personal observations in life as well such as when my parents dealt with my maternal grandfather's illness. I was a young teenager and didn't understand the impact at the time but later in life I could reflect on the energy, financial burdens and sacrifice they endured being concerned caregivers to a dying parent. Because they lived in Florida and my grandparents in Tennessee, they had to endure the burden of long distance, not being able to be there every day. I've had many conversations with caregivers of sarcoidosis patients, or people who must take care of their aging parents or grandparents and read many stories relating to both situations of dealing with loved ones with chronic health conditions and aging.

My primary observations came by watching my wife take care of me from the time we met until today as my health influences our every move. I watch as she handles her other responsibilities while at the same time knowing at any time I could need her uninterrupted attention. With that experience I made sure I always speak up for all caregivers. I want everyone, especially chronically ill patients, to understand what a difficult responsibility being a primary caregiver is and to appreciate all our loved ones do for us. But like I've said many times over, "You can never truly understand how someone or something feels unless you experience it for yourself, and even then we're all still unique individuals, but at least you have a firsthand knowledge of how that experience and responsibility feels."

For me the firsthand experience of understanding the physical, mental and emotional aspects of being a primary caregiver for a loved one with a health condition started in late 2002 when my wife was diagnosed with cancer. I remember the day she was diagnosed like it was yesterday. The emotions are overwhelming as the only thing we seemed to be able to do was cry, together and alone. I tried to maintain strength but in this situation the emotions were overwhelming. She was only 39 years old and had her whole life ahead of her. Anger, self-pity, frustration, fear of the unknown and even guilt that she had cancer when it should have been me all ran amok inside of me. She was the backbone of the family and to even have the possibility she might not be with us much longer scared the hell out of me. Let me tell you something; I've dealt with the frustrations of the unknown as I live with sarcoidosis and past doctors have mentioned my own death as a possibility to me, both past, present, and future, but there isn't anything scarier in this world than having a loved one told they have cancer! The word itself stirs so many emotions in an individual.

I felt helpless beyond explanation. I could deal with my own health and fate without much trouble but for my wife to be facing an uphill battle that could have unthinkable consequences and impact on my life was harder than I had ever imagined. After a couple of weeks we had cried all we could cry thus my wife took the attitude, as the strong woman she is, enough is enough, let's take care of this problem.

The one thing I've never had a problem with is discussing the positives and negatives of a situation. I feel both sides need to be discussed so you can prepare for any result. If you can deal with the most positive result and the most negative you should in turn be able to deal with anything in between. I must admit for the first time in my life preparing for the negative in this case was too much for me. Losing Ma-Shelle to death would have been like losing a part of my heart and soul. It was not something I even wanted to consider.

Around this time we had bought a house and were going to move from our downtown Detroit high-rise apartment to a house just outside the city. I think the hustle of going though the process of buying a house and getting it move-in ready increased the stress. Although the moving process is stressful in itself, at least it gave us something else to worry about even though in reality the fact cancer was in my wife's body weighed heavily on both of us, not to mention our 19-year-old daughter.

The decision was made to have surgery to attempt to remove the cancer. The surgery was scheduled the first week of March 2003. I have never felt so helpless and scared as I did during the four and a half hour surgery! I remember the cold feeling I felt inside as I watched her walk away not knowing if this would be the last time I ever saw her alive or in good health. It doesn't matter how simple the surgery is, anytime you put someone under there are possibilities for tragic consequences and this was no simple surgery by any length of anyone's imagination. I had done all the praying and mental preparation I could do and I knew she had a good team of doctors, but still the reality of there was nothing I could do tore me up inside. I went straight to the restroom and prayed one more time as I cried. With the guidance of God, she pulled through the surgery with flying colors!

We ended up physically moving on the day after she was released from the hospital, which is a story of its own. I was scheduled to speak at a conference in Los Angeles the next weekend. This was a commitment I'd made about eight months prior to someone who had been very supportive of me, therefore I wanted to do all I could to keep it. On that Wednesday we were about to go for a follow-up when she noticed an infection in her wound. As I was sitting in the waiting room the nurse came and called me back to the examining room. They had taken out most of the 50 plus staples and had the open wound exposed. The nurse proceeded to tell us we were going to have to clean the wound several times a day and wanted me to see what needed to take place. Knowing my fear of needles, or actually in this case more so it was the image of something going in the way a needle does, my wife had a mischievous look in her eyes as she gave me a little smile.

The nurse started by showing me how deep the wound was by sticking one of those long Q-tips into the wound. I made it through that little demonstration although I had to force myself to watch. I'm the primary caregiver in this situation so I have to be strong, or at least that's what I kept telling myself. I was feeling so-so, although I was starting to yawn repeatedly (my brain was trying to get oxygen I was later told) and felt a little tingly as the nurse showed us the first step, which was to clean the wound by pouring a fluid directly into the wound. I knew I didn't like this at all and was getting kind of hot inside as well. Then it was time to pack the wound. The nurse took out a bandage and wrapped it around another long Q-tip then stuck the Q-tip into the wound and pushed the bandage down inside the wound. That was my last straw!

The next thing I knew I started feeling intense heat inside my body and became very lightheaded, as I looked away from what the nurse was doing. "Are you okay?" I heard my wife ask, as I looked up at her and now understood the mischievous look in her eyes, as she knew what my reaction would most likely be. The next thing I knew the doctor had me in a wheelchair pushing me outside to cool off in the 20-degree Detroit morning weather. After a short while I was back to normal. Fortunately for me, when I returned to the room the wound had been covered and my wife said she would be able to do the procedure herself, as long as I could hold a mirror for her while hiding behind it and not watch what she was doing. We found a place for her to set the mirror and she was able to do the process herself. I flew to Los Angeles that Friday, kept my commitment and returned Sunday. Thank God she was a strong independent woman! Okay, you can stop laughing at me anytime now.

Here's the kicker…what if she hadn't been able to do the process alone? As the primary caregiver it was my responsibility and my responsibility alone to ensure the process was done on a regular basis. It was a safe statement to make I wasn't going to be able to do it myself. I would have done her more harm by maybe passing out with the Q-Tip in her wound or who knows what else. However the reality was my phobia didn't matter. All that mattered was getting the required process done. That was my responsibility!

As the primary caregiver there will be many times you must do things you don't want to do. This is just a fact of life when it comes to being a caregiver. The stress can be overwhelming at times but it's your responsibility to do whatever it takes, by any means necessary, to ensure the patient receives the proper care he/she needs. If you can't do it yourself you must find other ways to get it done. You have no other choice! Step out of your square, swallow your pride, make a million calls, research resources, but do what must be done, whatever that may be. I now understood this requirement more than ever.

I'm proud to say that as of 2009, Ma-Shelle is still cancer free and can declare herself an official cancer survivor. I felt I had a better understanding of what she went through with me and was just glad my role of primary caregiver was over. As fate would have it in the fall of 2003 my mother-in-law was diagnosed too with cancer and the role of team caregiver now started.

The difference in this situation for me wasn't emotional or mental because those feelings remained the same, although on a different emotional level. It was the physical responsibilities that were different. My wife took over the role of primary caregiver and even though her health was still technically in recovery and my health always remains an issue, the role of caregivers was now at the forefront. My mother-in-law went through a long surgery but radiation and chemotherapy was also going to be required. I took the role of the person who took her to chemotherapy and sat with her throughout the process.

It was actually a good feeling inside to know I was able to be there for my mother-in-law instead of always having people being concerned about me. It wasn't easy and at times hard on me healthwise as well because, after all, just because I'm helping others doesn't mean my health problems take a vacation. No, unlike other professions, as a "Professional Patient" you get no vacations!

There were many times when I had to fight through my own health issues to uphold my responsibilities, such as the example earlier where I took my wife to the ER then immediately took my mother-in-law to her appointments. As a caregiver there's no room for "I don't feel like it today." Everyday is your responsibility! The important thing to remember is you must understand your body and the limit for which you can successfully act as a caregiver. If you can't do something then it's your responsibility to ensure your responsibility is covered. I now understood the tremendous pressure you can feel as a caregiver.

In reality you, as a chronically ill patient yourself, can only go the extreme on a strictly when needed basis. It's critical everyone, even more so for someone who battles chronic health conditions, always keep your own health in the front of your thinking process, without guilt. After all if I didn't manage my own health I wouldn't be of any value to my mother-in-law or wife. You have to always be aware of your body signs and be honest with what you can and can't do healthwise to ensure you don't make commitments you can't keep or else find alternate options. A thin line to walk but you must be honest with yourself and loved ones during every step in order to successfully reach the final destination!

Aside from the chemotherapy duties my real responsibilities from this situation was to ease the burden on my wife. I had to step up and take care of other areas of our life including doing things for her grandmother, whom she was primarily taking care of at this time as well. There's so much more to life than the obvious and as team caregivers it was critical all areas were covered. Of course the physical demands, still combined with the mental and emotional feelings involved with supporting a loved one, especially when cancer is involved, still existed. I had learned a lot about being a caregiver and regardless of what I thought before it was a lot more difficult when you wore the caregiver hat. I sure had a renewed respect for what my wife and other caregivers had to endure. Together we got through it and it looked like I was two for two when it came to getting loved ones through the battles of cancer.

The only thing is you can't control fate and as fate would have it for the third time, I was about to understand firsthand yet another scenario of being a caregiver. In May 2004 my father, a lifelong smoker, was diagnosed with lung cancer in addition to a severe case of emphysema. Since he was too old (77) to survive surgery and chemotherapy was not a vital option for his type of cancer and age, the treatments were going to consist of six to seven weeks of radiation. My father still lived in Perry, a rural town in Florida about an hour south of Tallahassee, which is where the radiation treatments were to take place. Basically he would have an hour drive to the cancer center, about 30 minutes or so for the treatments, then another hour ride home along with about 30 minutes to and from the hospital once in Tallahassee. The treatments would be everyday, Monday through Friday. In June I dropped everything and flew to Florida so I could drive him to and from his treatments, leaving our family responsibilities to Ma-Shelle as in this scenario she took the indirect caregiver role and was now the one responsible for not only her normal tasks but mine as well. I remember the first thing she said to me when I told her he was diagnosed with cancer. She looked me directly in the eyes and asked, "When are you leaving?" Without hesitation we both knew what had to be done.

From an emotional standpoint, although you really can't truly compare the situations fairly, I think my wife's diagnosis probably shook and shocked me the most, especially from an emotional standpoint.

With my father, in the back of my mind, his being diagnosed with lung cancer after smoking over a pack a day for over 50 years, after the initial normal emotional reaction was over, was not shocking. No one who smokes cigarettes is immune to lung cancer! I'll say this, without a doubt this situation was the most demanding from a physical perspective.

For one my father had never been sick to amount to anything in his life and now he was not only diagnosed with the scariest word a patient could hear, "cancer", but he was having to deal with doctor appointment after doctor appointment and waiting, waiting and more waiting. This was a process, as described earlier, that required major adjustments on his part both physically and mentally, not to mention the enormous stress it created for him on a minute-to-minute basis.

There was all of the paperwork to deal with as well. He had insurance paperwork, each individual doctor's paperwork, each individual test or labs paperwork, emergency room paperwork, the American Cancer Society's paperwork (they have excellent benefits such as reimbursement for gas to and from treatments, so always look into what you might be entitled to), medical equipment paperwork, as the list went on and on. Having to keep him calm and anxiety as low as possible plus ensure all of the paperwork was done correctly took an enormous amount of energy, which at times was hard to find. As always my health conditions don't go away just because I'm needed elsewhere. Add the additional stress of being away from my wife and normal routine, including my own bed, for a long length of time on the spur of the moment all took a personal toll on me, both physically and mentally. Don't try and read between the lines or falsely interpret what I'm saying because make no mistake about it I'm not complaining nor looking for a gold star. You do what's right without question and as I stated earlier all children have an unconditional obligation to care for their parents when needed, especially when their father had done for them in the positive manner mine had done for me my entire life. If the situation repeated itself tomorrow I would be in Florida today without hesitation! With that said…reality is still reality!

There was another factor that came into play in this situation as well…my mother. My parents had one of those storybook marriages. They were married in 1947 and I never saw them have a serious argument or be sincerely mad at each other for any measurable length of time. Ask my mother and she can't remember a situation either. To be honest this isn't as good for the child as it might seem since it gave me an unrealistic view of relationships. All relationships have conflict and there's a right and wrong way to deal with conflict. I had to learn the right way over the years; therefore I feel it's important to let your children understand conflict is normal, just teach them the proper way to deal with it. Another thing is my mother had never spent more than a few nights away from him the entire time they had been married. In fact, and I swear this is true, she had never spent a night alone her entire life, as a kid, teenager, or adult. If she was away from him she was with other people or visiting us in Detroit. Just imagine the emotions she must have felt regarding the uncertainty of what life would be like without her husband. Even when my father spent the night in the hospital she stayed by his side the entire night. Storybook!

Like my father, my mother was a lifelong teacher, now retired, and worked part-time at a local dress store. She has one of the most positive attitudes about life you will ever encounter. No matter what you tell her about anything she'll find something positive to say about it. She is also very outgoing. Sit by her for a minute and before you know it you'll be in a conversation, and if you stay there for very long you'll know a lot about her and she'll know a lot about you. She's nonstop from the time she wakes up until the time she lies on the sofa to watch television, with her eyes closed, that evening. She just can't stay still and relax, as she will say, "There is always something that needs to be done." More than anything she's a sincere, caring and strong woman.

From my perspective I felt I needed to pay almost as much attention to her as to my father. If she burned herself out she wasn't going to be able to withstand the long journey my father was about to travel. She had been there for her parents but at the time she was younger and they were long distance. Having her husband in a life-threatening situation, regardless of how positive she was on the outside, I know tore her up inside. At least she had her sister and her husband, who are wonderful people, along with many friends to help her out, an advantage of living in a small town. However all of that didn't help me when it came to my concerns about her well being, as the helplessness weighed heavily on my mind.

It was hard at times getting him to do the things he was supposed to do and help him battle the mind games of dealing with cancer when you've never been sick. The everyday routines he had done for years were changing and change was not something he adjusted to very well, in the beginning. However, to everyone's surprise, the last months of his life he accepted with dignity changes such as giving up golf and driving, as he went with the flow his ever changing health dictated for him. But for me it was something I had never dealt with in this manner before, and I remember I kept thinking again and again of how my wife had handled me and her other responsibilities all these years, as my appreciation and respect for not only her but all caregivers continued to increase dramatically.

I was able to build a good relationship with his doctor and the specialists. My father was not the best patient or easiest to deal with and at times didn't understand the reality of being sick. He just could never grasp the concept he wasn't the most important patient the doctor had. There were times when tough love had to come into play. I remember one time he was supposed to be drinking Gatorade, but wouldn't, so as a direct result he developed dehydration problems. We kept telling him to drink his Gatorade but he refused to do it. It got to the point where he had to go to the doctor for a couple of days and have an IV for about three hours in order to get liquid directly into his body. He actually seemed to look forward to having to go the first time as he said when my mother tried to get him to drink some Gatorade, "I'll just go to the doctor and they'll give me an IV while I watch golf on television and visit." See what I mean? He just didn't seem to get the reality of being sick and for his own good it was time to put a stop to this hotel/vacation mentality before it cost him his life or the crying wolf theory became his reputation. We already know the danger in that.

I went to the doctor with him to drop him off and discreetly asked if I could speak to the doctor privately first while he was getting setup with his IV. When we were alone I told the doctor, "I think we've built a good relationship between us, plus you've read my book so I think you understand my point of views, therefore I hope you take this the way it's intended. My father seems to think this is a vacation or something and doesn't take it for the seriousness it is. His attitude is I can just come over here, get my IV and watch golf." The doctor shook his head in agreement; after all doctors can pickup on the crying wolf theory or denial factor better than patients think. I continued, "For my father's own good I want you to do me a favor. When you give him the IV, for whatever reason you can think of, make sure your television isn't working today. Without causing him any harm I want him to be bored out of his head and not want to ever have to come here for an IV when he can simply drink his Gatorade at home. This is one procedure that's avoidable." "Don't worry, I totally agree and I got you covered", the doctor replied. We shook hands and I left my father in his care.

When I returned a few hours later my father was ready to get home. On the ride home he kept complaining the cable was out and after he sat down no one paid any attention to him, as they were so busy. "I dread having to go over there again tomorrow", he snapped. "If you would drink your Gatorade like you're supposed to you wouldn't have to", I replied without sympathy. When we got home in a caring tone I told him, "If you want me to I'll go to Wal*Mart and get you different flavors of Gatorade or anything else you might like to drink. Carnation Instant Breakfast was something I used to drink when I was sick and didn't have an appetite. Maybe you would like to try that too." He spent the next day at the doctor's office bored, as once again the cable was out. However from then on he did exactly what he was supposed to do in regard to drinking his Gatorade and didn't have a dehydration problem again. As a caregiver sometimes you have to understand when to give tough love and when to cater to the patient's needs, or both. It's a thin line but one each caregiver must learn for each individual patient as, like with the grieving process, we are all unique individuals when it comes to dealing with our health.

Eventually and with a lot of up and down times we made it through the treatments successfully. It looked as if the cancer was under control so it was time for me to go back to Detroit. Having a parent or loved one you feel needs your daily support living so far away can be a very stressful mental battle on a daily basis. When I returned home, up until the time he passed, I called home every single day regardless of where I was. It became a part of my daily life that up until now had not existed. After I moved out and lived on my own I had only talked to my parents primarily on Wednesdays and Sundays, any other time something was probably wrong or it was a holiday. It wasn't that we weren't close but neither my father nor I were phone talkers. Of course for my mother that wasn't the case as she could talk on the phone or in person anytime of the day or night. She had gotten in the Wednesday/Sunday habit with her mother so it just kind of transferred to us when I moved away. After my father's death I still try to call my mother on a daily basis just to let her know I'm always just a phone call away.

This was also the first time my father started telling me he loved me on a regular basis when we would hang up. Although his love was never questioned, as I was the most loved child on this earth, he just wasn't one for emotional words like that between us. I guess it was just another of those male ego things. He showed his love by his actions not words.

Having a health condition that could take or alter your life makes you look at things in your life a little differently. It's no different for the caregiver. I couldn't imagine, although you understand all things must eventually come to an end, not having my wife, mother-in-law or father around. You really start to appreciate the little things more and more. It's sad something has to happen that threatens the existence of a person or relationship to make you again appreciate what made that person or relationship special. It happens to us all in various ways. Try not to put yourself in that situation and appreciate each and every day, as if it were your last.

Things were going along pretty good although being away was hard because you can only do so much, and you're dependent on others telling you the truth about what's going on. I understand most of us will hold back because we don't want to worry a person we love who couldn't do anything about the daily situation anyway. As a patient I've done it on more than one occasion, so who am I to talk? Your perspective sure changes when you're the loved one worrying at a long distance, dependent on others for statuses, as the helplessness starts to become a daily companion. I never truly knew what to believe, as my father didn't want to worry me and my mother is so damn positive, although towards the end she became more open. I was learning the true meaning and consequences of helplessness!

In February 2005 I flew back to Florida as my father was going to have surgery to put stints in his legs and have his arteries cleared of blockage. He had had this surgery for his arteries earlier, and I found out while listening to conversations they thought he had died during recovery, something I had never been told. This only made my stress level go up as my faith in being told the whole truth when I returned to Detroit just became more suspect. He came through the surgery in flying colors so I returned home where I continued my daily calls.

In April 2005 I got more troubling news. During his routine follow-ups it was suspected something was wrong with his bladder. After further tests it was concluded cancer had spread to his bladder. Radiation was again going to be the treatment. This time I didn't want to depend on information from my mother, as her information seemed to change slightly each time we talked. It was no fault of hers or malicious intentions; its just there was so much to comprehend she, at times, got confused and understandably so.

Since I was on my father's HIPAA sheet, I called the doctor direct. I was able to talk to a nurse who gave me the straight facts as she read me the doctor's actual notes. It seemed it was too dangerous to give him the dosage of radiation needed to kill the tumor directly; accordingly they were going to treat the area around the bladder to build a fence of types so the cancer couldn't spread. This method should allow him some extra time and a better quality of life. Although this type of news causes emotional depression, I appreciated her honesty. I strongly believe in dealing with the truth head on; therefore, I always want to know exactly what I am facing, whether as a patient or a caregiver.

I flew to Florida the day before Mother's Day to take him to his radiation treatments and planned on staying until after Father's Day. This time around he was calmer and seemed to have adjusted somewhat to being a cancer patient. This dosage and location didn't have the side effects as the previous treatments and overall he handled the situation well. For me the helplessness still weighed strong because I knew we were only preventing the cancer from spreading and not killing it. As a caregiver I had to control my emotions so I could take care of him and ensure my mother got a break from the everyday care she was providing while I was in Detroit. My concern for her well being was still as great, if not greater, than my concern for my father. Now more than ever I understood the patient can deal with the situation a lot better than a loved one in the role of caregiver, whether it be in the role of primary or long distance. For myself, I must admit, this situation was hard and as always I looked to my Faith for inner strength. I continued to deal with my own health situations, which were more difficult on a daily basis with the additional stress of being a long distance caregiver. But, you do what you have to do!

Back in Detroit another problem arose. My mother-in-law was having problems with a persistent cough and movement in her right arm. While watching a newscast regarding lung cancer and persistent coughing my wife urged her to make an appointment with her doctor. The results from her chest X-ray came back abnormal with suspicion of cancer. As a result of our bonding during her last bout with radiation and chemotherapy she kept asking when I was coming home. I talked to her on the phone several times ensuring her I would be there for her during any treatments and like the last time we would kick cancer's butt. At this time in my life I felt closer to my mother-in-law than ever before!

When she went for her follow-up appointment, her doctor took one look at her arm, immediately gave her a voucher for a cab and sent her to the hospital. It turned out cancer was in her bones, as well as her lungs and other parts of her body, causing the bone in her arm to be completely severed. As much pain as I have endured and endure on a daily basis, I can't even begin to comprehend the pain she was experiencing with every movement. As with my father, round two was getting ready to start and the roll of caregiver was getting harder and harder to endure as I felt pulled from all angles, which continued to cause a negative impact on my own health. Right or wrong, I kept quiet about my personal issues because at this time my health, unless critical, was not the primary focus nor could it be a distraction. I understood my body to the extent I knew what I could and couldn't do and also recognized the impact of my actions on my mother-in-law, father, and wife. I also had faith God wouldn't give me too much to handle.

My father's treatment ended, however I decided to cut my visit short and fly back to Detroit to be with my mother-in-law and wife. We went to see the bone specialist and while he was reading her report I could tell by the look on his face she was in bad shape, as he took a deep breath and turned to face us (he wasn't aware I could see his face while he read her report). He gave us the surgery options to repair her arm and we proceeded to schedule the surgery. In addition we met with her oncologist and decided to put off the chemotherapy until after the surgery to repair the severed bone in her arm.

We decided it was best for her to come stay with us so we brought her to our home where, my wife primarily and I as the indirect, could take better care of her. It was the best decision we could have made as it gave us both a chance to bond even closer with her and learn things about her we never knew. For us it was a no brainier, but for some having a loved one move into your home can be a hard decision. With that decision comes a complete change to your everyday life. Taking care of a sick loved one, causes everything in your daily life to change, especially someone who is basically dependent on you. It's a responsibility of tremendous impact on your family from a physical, mental and financial standpoint, but to us, it wasn't a decision at all but an unconditional obligation. For us the logic is simple…you do what you have to do and no pat on the back is expected.

No one should judge anyone, but for some the responsibility of becoming a caregiver is too much to handle. If the responsibility is too much, ask for help while doing what you can, as that's part of being a successful caregiver as well. Just be honest about your intentions. You have to live with yourself, and you might only have this opportunity to care for your loved one to the best of your ability. From experience I would advise you to do whatever is necessary to care for your loved ones because once it's too late you don't want to live with the guilt of what you should have done, knowing you were thinking only of yourself. I've seen the result of guilt and it's not a pretty sight!

The first day of the surgery the surgeon was running late so the surgery was postponed. This was the hand of God because it gave her son the opportunity he wouldn't have otherwise had to bring her grandchildren to visit, as he lived in Utah. We had a big fish fry at our house and I believe it gave her a wonderful feeling to have all of her loved ones by her side even though she was obviously in tremendous pain. On the day of the next surgery attempt it was determined at the last minute if she was put under and had to lie flat, the position required for the surgery, she would not make it through the surgery. This was determined based on the current stage of the cancer in her lungs. Therefore the decision was made to have her do a couple of chemotherapy treatments then do the surgery. I still can't even begin to imagine the pain she had to be in with a severed bone in her arm.

Two days before her first chemotherapy treatment was to be performed, a Wednesday, she fell onto the bed, as she came from the restroom, and broke her hip. This resulted in a no choice decision, although the same danger was still present, to perform surgery to repair the hip. The surgery was performed on Friday, July 8, 2005. She passed away peacefully surrounded by family and friends on Sunday, July 10, 2005. The last words I said to her Saturday night were, "See you later. I love you."

During all of this my father was hospitalized in Florida with pneumonia. After my mother-in-law's funeral we drove to Florida to see him and hopefully the drive down Interstate 75 through the mountains would allow us to relax and, at least for a couple of days, take a break from the stress we had been dealing with as caregivers and deal with our individual grief as well. I knew deep down my father's journey had reached the final stretch.

Two appointments were scheduled, one with the urologist for his bladder and later with the oncologist for his lungs. We took my father to Tallahassee in hopes of a good report and to find out why the pneumonia wouldn't clear up. The first stop was with the urologist and to everyone's surprise the cancer had disappeared. Even though the purpose of the radiation treatment was to build a fence to contain the cancer in the bladder, it had cured itself, or in my mind escaped. As the doctor put it, "Your bladder looks 200% better and is cancer free!" We couldn't have been happier and we were all riding on cloud nine, although I must admit my inner voice was telling me not to get too excited. Next we were off to the oncologist.

My inner voice was correct, as I knew something wasn't right when the doctor left the room to compare his current X-rays with his most recent and stayed gone for quite a while. When he returned the news was not what we wanted to hear. The reason for the pneumonia was a result of cancer aggressively returning to his lungs. We had four options but only one was realistic. We had done all of the radiation the lungs could take. Chemotherapy was too dangerous, as was surgery. Therefore the only option we had was to manage the symptoms. In other words make my father's quality of life the best it could be because as far as the cancer, it was too far gone to treat.

My father took the news, especially compared to how he was in the beginning of this journey, extremely well. My mother on the other hand took it hard. She is an extremely strong woman but once she breaks, she breaks, and I personally believe the stress from all of the care she had provided on a daily basis since the beginning of this journey finally got to her. For me the hardest thing in the world is to see my wife, daughter or mother cry when there's nothing I can do to ease their pain. The helplessness at this point in time was extreme. I did all I could to stay strong, the need to be the strong male figure in me coming out, until I was in private where I too broke down from the news. In addition I was still grieving from my mother-in-law's recent passing, as I had tried to be the strong male support figure for my wife and daughter the past few weeks. My heart was also heavy for my wife, as I knew she was in tremendous pain as well. In private I just couldn't be strong any longer!

As we left for Detroit I think it was the hardest time in my life I ever had to say goodbye to my parents, not knowing if this was realistically the last time I would ever see my father alive. The next week on August 1, 2005, home hospice, a wonderful service, came and took over, providing everything he and my mother needed. After the initial overwhelming of emotions, going for a routine follow-up appointment to being told death was intimate to your home being completely uprooted, life calmed down, my father adjusted well to his new fate. He continued to accept his changing situation up until his death better than any of us would have imagined.

For me as a long distance caregiver, it was hard. I was still dealing with grieving my mother-in-law's death, my wife's grief, and the uncertainty of my father's fate, plus our daughter was expecting our first granddaughter, a different role as grandfather was beginning as well. Of course you can never forget the impact my own health issues had on me as my diabetes mellitus was getting worse, and the possibility of going on insulin scared the hell out of me.

I still called Florida everyday but my heart would skip a beat every time they called me. I was scared to answer the phone when their number popped up on my caller id. Not knowing if I should return to visit, not knowing what I could do, but worrying about my mother overdoing it, understanding the stress she was under with me a thousand miles away took a toll on my health and mental outlook. Learning to deal with this situation took a lot of soul searching. The one thing I did make sure of is I didn't do anything, or not do anything, that would allow guilt to be in my future.

As it was with my mother-in-law staying with us, I felt I became closer to my father during our daily phone calls. We are who we are so it's not like we talked for hours. Just hearing his voice and helping him out with questions he might have made me feel a little useful.

I still was able to visit him a few times before his death and I could tell little differences when I saw him in person I wasn't able to notice on the phone. I know it was difficult for my mother and I worried about her constantly. You can have all the support in the world but the reality is sometime during the day or when you lie down at night you're alone and you must find a way to deal with your emotions. In April 2006 my father passed away.

The last thing I ever said to him was, "I love you and I'll be careful." He would always say, "be careful" to me when I would leave the house and it bugged the heck out of me. For some reason I said that to him when I left the hospice room that night. I think deep down I knew this was his last night.

In my father's case, I was prepared for his death. What I was going to do, how I was going to handle the different situations, the funeral and my overall grieving process. The reality is, in any situation, you can't prepare for how you're going to react to a loved ones death. You might think you can, but when reality hits, it hits each situation and us all differently. Although I might not show it on the outside and I'm still waiting for the unexpected moment when I can cry the internal grief away, my father's death hurts tremendously and I miss him greatly!

I stayed in Florida for a month or so helping my mother with all of the other issues that arise from death. She did very good as we got rid of all his clothes, changed financial policies, and a multitude of other things you don't think about until you're faced with the tasks. Finally it was time for me to go back to Detroit and for my mother to spend the first night of her life alone. I remember driving the 18-hour journey, primarily in rain, back to Detroit in one day. For the first time in my life I couldn't bare being alone that night.

As time passed she has handled the grieving process well. Hospice came by a few times to follow-up on her and she has a lot of support from friends and family. I know she has her bad moments but overall I'm proud of her strength and the way she continues to live life. It doesn't matter who you are we all must go at some point in time and after we're gone life will continue for those we leave behind. Death is a fact of life we all must come to terms with at some point in our lives.

Something else I'm extremely proud of is the fact my father, mother or anyone else never blamed anyone else for my father's fate. I know this will probably tick some of you off; therefore let me first say I was a smoker myself. My father smoked exposing me to second hand smoke my entire childhood and teenage years, and my father died as a direct result of smoking cigarettes; thus I have the right to make these statements, like it or not. Smokers and their families need to understand when people smoke and expose their loved ones to secondhand smoke it's by their own choice. Everyone knows the dangers of smoking; therefore please stop blaming the tobacco industry for the fact your loved one died from smoking and you were exposed to secondhand smoke. Take responsibility for yourself and hold your loved one responsible for choosing to smoke…period.

I very seldom defend corporate America and I'm not defending the tobacco industry now. I feel it's terrible an industry can legally sell a product that kills. The tobacco industry also has the best marketing teams around. It's amazing to me the PR they have and confidence in the fact people are going to smoke regardless of what they say or the programs they're forced to create. Think about this for a second. The tobacco industry will tell you not to start smoking. However if you do, then we have the best cigarettes for you. When you've finally reached the point where you're either tired of smoking, the cigarettes have caused you financial issues, since they aren't cheap, or your health is at the point you have to stop, we'll tell you how to quit and even help you. What other product would have the confidence and at the same time be so hypocritical to be able to make these promises. You have to look closely at most advertising and programs to see the subliminal methods and hypocrisy with which the tobacco industry pushes their products (that again are proven to kill). Most are under the corporate name and tobacco or cigarettes aren't included.

The other thing is our elected officials allow a product that is proven to kill to be sold legally in America. There is no proven benefit to smoking tobacco. People die as a direct result of smoking cigarettes everyday and it's not an easy or cheap death. In fact it's the taxpayers who a lot of times end up funding the bill, such as with Medicare, for those who die a slow death from smoking a legally killing product. The rules for exposing what's in cigarettes aren't even the same as our food, which doesn't kill you. What's wrong with this picture?

The bottom line is the person chose to smoke regardless of the known danger. I started smoking in fifth grade and I knew the danger then. That was probably part of the thrill, along with the cool television commercials that showed during that time in history. So stop the lawsuits, even though a lot of money has been rewarded, a majority of which went to the lawyers. The greed and overcrowding of the courts have caused a multitude of others who have been wrongfully treated of no fault of theirs to extend their suffering while the court system struggles to meet the demand of their case loads. It was the responsibility of the individual for choosing to smoke and if your loved one exposed you to secondhand smoke it was their responsibility, not someone else. It is what it is.

That's why I'm proud not one single person even mentioned the fact it was anyone's fault my father smoked his entire life other than my father's. My father enjoyed his cigarettes. Like all of the other smokers it was his choice. Life is what it is and sometimes you just have to accept the free actions of those you love and move on with the consequences. This is one of those situations!

From a personal perspective I don't know which is easier (for lack of a better term) to deal with as a survivor, the instant death, the short-term illness leading to death or the long-term long distance process leading to death. I've experienced each scenario with three individuals who were all an important part of my life, physically and emotionally. In the end the process in which they passed didn't matter. It was the individual whom I miss and each situation required a time of grief.

A caregiver's responsibilities are many and as a chronically ill patient yourself you must never forget about your own health, without guilt. No one can take care of another if you can't take care of yourself. This is even truer for a chronically ill patient turned caregiver. Caregivers have the responsibility to watch the patient's back and be their eyes, ears and sometimes mind. A caregiver must understand the patient's situation and desires because it might come down to the caregiver to make tough decisions such as do you want life support if that time comes. As always honest communications about the tough subjects need to be discussed beforehand because there's no second-guessing when reality hits. Never forget reality can hit at any moment. Be prepared as best as you can.

Each individual is different and has different desires. I know one of the hardest things for me as a caregiver was understanding and accepting the different ways my loved ones handled their own health processes, even though I understood it was a necessity. All of them from my wife to my mother-in-law to my father were completely different and all handled their health situation as a patient in many ways differently from how I wanted them to do things. I can write about it all day from a patient's perspective but it takes experiencing life in the shoes of a caregiver to truly understand and appreciate the self-control it takes to pull off caring for a loved one successfully. The reality is it must be pulled off successfully because individuals must deal with their own health situation their individual way, not the caregiver's way. For a caregiver this is probably the toughest thing to understand, accept and accomplish. To take it one step further as a patient who deals with living with chronic health conditions every day of my life, I felt I had the experience and knowledge to guide each of them through their battles in the manner that was best for me. Understanding, and even more so, accepting that my way wasn't always the best way was indescribably difficult for me.

You must walk a fine line between letting the patient deal with his/her health needs and stepping in when their way isn't working, without fear of guilt or resentment as a result of your decisions. Being a caregiver under any circumstance is hard; therefore please do what you must to understand and accept this fact of life so you can better deal with all of the responsibilities and emotions you're going to experience. Patients and loved ones need their caregivers! Regardless of the reaction of the patient, who might not be in their right frame of mind, always remember your value and responsibilities.

...11...

There are times in life when you must put your personal issues aside for those you love and as a result face possible personal, financial, or health hardships. At the same time you must never put your health in jeopardy. In turn don't expect a gold star but instead just remember, "If you do right, right will come back to you!"

12

Understanding Insurance Is The Difference

I have a question. Couldn't, in 21st century America, insurance just be another name for legal racketeering? Wait a minute now, you might say, that's an off the wall question! Let's take a closer look at the possibilities. What is racketeering? Racketeering is usually described as *"one who obtains money illegally in exchange for protection from harm, usually by intimidation"*. If we exchange the word illegally for legally don't we have insurance? In fact isn't insurance what the racketeers called their "services"?

We're setup in this society where there's very little we can get, of value, without insurance. Try buying a house or getting a mortgage without insurance…can't be done. Try buying a car or getting a license plate without insurance…can't be done. Insurance isn't an option it's mandatory. Once you pay for the protection and the right to have the home or car, and nothing happens and you don't need to use the insurance, you don't get any of the money back, do you? Even many apartment managements will require you to purchase rental insurance on your property, not theirs, in order to rent an apartment. Not an op-tion or of any value to the apartment management, that I can see, but a requirement nonetheless in order for you to rent an apartment.

What about when you have to use it? It can be an intimidating process where you're discouraged not to file a claim or you come to find out in the fine print you aren't covered anyway. Your agent, or the documentation misleads you when you were buying the policy or the fine print was too much for the average person to comprehend. Don't believe me? Ask the victims of Hurricane Katrina who paid insurance policies for years thinking the protection they were paying for was there when they needed it! And why is it, does our next premium always go up when we file a claim? It doesn't go down, if we don't. After a home invasion in 2006 my homeowners' insurance went from $1,200 a year to $2,500. Needless to say I switched to another company who gave me the same coverage for $900 a year.

On the flip side why do businesses such as medical professionals, auto repair shops, and home repair businesses; to name a few, charge a higher price for work in which insurance claims are filed and a lower price for the same work performed for customers without an insurance claim? Remember my chiropractor who immediately went from his $88 insurance fee to a $44 charge for me since I didn't have insurance. I see commercials for auto paint shops and body shops that use this method all the time to get accident customers. If the job requires the same supplies, the same amount of work, and the same amount of time to complete the job then why are the prices different?

The customer/policy holder suffers in the end when an insurance company is ripped off. Let's call it what it is because if they can perform the same task for a profit for someone without insurance then, in turn, by charging a higher price for the same work in order to get extra monies from an insurance company it is ripping them off. As with any business the more expenses a business has the higher their fees, or in this case premiums, will be in order to make up for the expenses. When it's all said and done they aren't doing anyone a favor but themselves.

Let's not forget the legislation that comes out after a disaster favoring the insurance industry and what they're required to pay, especially when the insurance industry complains about costs and reminds our elected officials of their contributions. As the explanation goes, they'll go bankrupt and that's bad for our economy. However, nobody worries about the policyholder going bankrupt in order to make their required insurance premiums, as the consumers' lack of funds impacts the economy even more so. Wonder why?

I don't know about you but to me that surely does sound a lot like legal racketeering! Anyway, now that I've got that little bit of personal peeve out of the way, let's talk about health care insurance, which is required in some fashion if you stand any chance of getting "quality" health care.

There are many types of health care insurance ranging from Health Maintenance Organizations (HMOs), Preferred Provider Organizations (PPOs), Medicare, Medicaid, private personal insurance policies, dental, vision, supplementary, long-term care, life and prescription drug coverage; to name a few. If you're fortunate enough to be employed full-time, your coverage options are usually provided via your employer with you paying a portion of the premium and cost, which is getting higher each year. You may also receive health care coverage from the government or maybe you can afford to pay for the policy yourself. In most cases you have the option to choose your plan and what's covered, with a cost associated with each option, at the beginning of the calendar year (January 1st) and your coverage will last without you having the ability to change your policy (except for life altering situations where you might can add or delete someone from the policy, but not change the coverage) until the end of the calendar year (December 31st).

With that fact in mind let's start with the most important thing you must do in order to ensure you receive the health care coverage you need and can afford…understand your policy beforehand! This might sound like another of those simple statements but understanding your insurance policy, whether it's your home, auto or health care policies is something you must do and it won't be easy. In reality insurance policies are legal contracts between you and your insurance provider and the policies are written in such a manner, with much of the importance in very fine print. There's a lot of documentation and a single word can change the meaning of the policy, consequently you must be very careful in understanding what you're reading and the interpretation as the insurance company sees it, not as you see it. In fact in some cases the insurance company doesn't even have to provide you with all of the details upfront.

In 2002 I went to have my DDAVP refilled and found that in order to get the brand name as opposed to the generic version I was going to have to pay a calculation that read "brand name cost minus generic version cost plus $7". I looked at all the documentation provided to me and nowhere was this calculation mentioned. The only thing mentioned was I paid $7 for generic versions, $15 for brand name and $30 for non-preferred brands (those drugs your insurance company doesn't want you to use because of…). The documentation stated that generic versions were preferred when available, but nowhere did it mention required or the calculation.

Since I got the coverage from my employer, the source that actually determines your coverage since the insurance companies will cover almost anything if you pay for it, I had them look for the calculation but they too couldn't find it in their documentation. Finally after a couple of months of frustration and using the generic version with little success, the insurance company provided the documentation to my employer with the requirement and calculation listed.

Turns out that year in Michigan the insurance company had 120 days after the policy was in affect to provide all of the documentation regarding what was actually covered to the policyholder…legally. My source of that legal information was my employer and health care provider, and I never received the calculation when determining my choice of coverage for the calendar year. Basically, without all of the documentation provided for me to make a logical decision I had picked a policy with coverage I could not change within the calendar year. Fortunately I filed an appeal and was able to get the brand name for the non-preferred price of $30 per month instead of the $120 per month. I received the rest of my documentation at home in April before the 120 day limit expired, and after I left the corporation on April 3rd, I was now on my wife's policy, same HMO but better coverage since it's again the corporation that determines your coverage. Does that actual scenario sound like the patient's rights are in the forefront to you? Be aware!

Another thing I've learned is the insurance company can change their pricing and what they cover, especially from a prescription drug standpoint, anytime during the calendar year, and yes you're still required to keep the same policy until December 31st. It happens all of the time and there's nothing you, the patient/policyholder/customer can do about it but pay it. Are you still wondering why I used the term legal racketeering?

The first step in understanding your policy beforehand is to gather all of the documentation you can get your hands on from your employer, government, and the insurance company. I know the documentation will be overwhelming at first but you must take the time to go through each and every piece of paper and/or screen online. If you have a family, it's important to get everyone involved because the more eyes you have the better chance you'll make a wise decision. Even get your children involved, to a certain degree, because an innocent child will ask very obvious, but logical questions that are too obvious to "us who know everything" adults.

Don't be afraid to ask questions as many times as needed to whomever you need to ask, be it your employer, insurance company or other individuals who have used the same coverage. There are a lot of things you must understand such as; (1) deductibles,(2) co-pays, (3) monthly cost, (4) emergency room cost , (5) prescription coverage, (6) dental coverage, and (7) vision coverage. Some of the other questions you need to ask are what doctors accept the coverage, are there any out of network costs, what are the processes to follow if you have problems or need to appeal, how to obtain referrals if needed, are there special accounts for emergency uses to contribute to with before taxes are taken out (although keep in mind in these cases if you don't use the funds you lose them), any limits on money you can use and hospital coverage. Keep in mind these are only a few of the basic information you need to find out as each of us have unique health care/insurance needs.

Secondly, you must look at your individual and family health care needs. Remember you won't get any money back just because you don't use a benefit. Sometimes you don't need a Cadillac when a bicycle will get you where you need to go. Keep in mind you can't predict your actual medical needs because at anytime your health can take a turn for the worse whether it be via an automobile accident or you develop a life altering disease. However in reality you can usually have a pretty good idea of your medical needs barring the unexpected. In my case, based on past experiences, I know I need the Cadillac because I have multiple chronic health conditions and can need emergency assistance at anytime. I need a multitude of prescription drugs on a daily basis to survive. I know my conditions are going to be with me for life so if anything my need for coverage will increase as opposed to decrease. Your case might be different and each individual case is what you should base your decision on. There should never be a "Keeping up with the Joneses" complex in regards to health care insurance.

Ask yourself some of these questions. Are you young and in good health? Do you use any prescription drugs? Do you anticipate any dental work coming up? How is your vision? Is anyone in your family expecting a child or wanting to become pregnant? Any minor or major surgeries expected? How has your health changed over the past year and do you anticipate the same progression this year? Do you have ample savings or other funds in case an emergency arises that's not covered? Are you willing and able to take the chance?

There are additional methods you can look at to save money as well. Some policies give discounts for non-smokers. Some discount if you belong to a health club or will provide a discount to join. There are programs for your diet, heart, diabetes, and others you can join in order to obtain possible discounts. Are their exercise programs your employer provides? Prevention is a major cost saver in the long run and some insurance companies and corporations are starting to understand it's cheaper to prevent health conditions and promote good health than treat the results of bad health habits. Ask your employer or insurance company for any details on ways you can save on your coverage because saving money is always on the top of the list for corporate America!

Once you have studied and understand all of the documentation to the best of your ability and have a comfortable prediction of your anticipated health care needs for the upcoming year, along with how you would pay for any unexpected health costs not covered, you're ready to make your choice. Don't think just because you've made your choice and now you're covered for the calendar year you don't have to stay on top of the situation and your coverage. Don't make that costly mistake! To the contrary, you're just now beginning.

One thing to keep in mind, as I mentioned earlier, your coverage can and will change in regard to pricing, specific drug coverage or procedures covered during your contract year. Although you're committed to the plan for the calendar year, your insurance company doesn't have the same rules. They can legally change parts of your policy and most times without notification to you until you try to use the policy or get a bill. Being prepared and aware of your coverage beforehand is of vital importance and a responsibility that falls on you the policyholder.

Before you have any procedure done discuss with your doctor's office, the medical facility or better yet, your insurance company to ensure you're covered. Usually your doctor isn't aware of your coverage, as their concern is your health. Some are up on the different policies but most don't have a clue regarding the specifics. It's hard enough staying on top of the changing medical procedures and health care treatment advances. This is why you must understand your coverage so when a doctor prescribes a medication, test or procedure you'll know if it's covered or at least have an idea of where to find out. If you aren't sure tell your doctor to check to see if you're covered (another reason to have a positive relationship with the staff) or else you check yourself. Either way find out before you get your test, lab work or procedure performed. It's you, the policyholder who is responsible once the work has been done to pay for anything not covered. Therefore spend the time beforehand while you don't owe anyone anything. Health care is no longer just what the doctor orders. Unfortunately we've gone beyond that reasonable logic.

In every doctor's office, lab or medical facility there's one sign hanging in a obvious place that reads something like this…"*It's the responsibility of the patient for payment of services rendered. Make sure if you have any insurance changes the staff is notified. All billing issues are between the patient and their insurance company, not the medical facility. Payment is due upon services rendered.*" Look around next time you're in any medical facility or doctor's office. It won't be hard to find. In fact it's usually hanging somewhere near where you sign in for your appointment or in the actual examining room. It will be right there in black and white stating you're responsible for all cost associated with your visit and if there are any issues with your insurance company that's between you and your insurance company. We expect our payment in full from you when services are rendered!

In today's medical environment it's your insurance that really determines your quality of health care, the majority of the time. Make sure you get the care to which you're entitled. Some policies allow certain tests to be performed only a certain number of times per year. Some require a preauthorization and explanation from your doctor before the procedure is approved. Some require you have a procedure done at a certain facility or else you pay a higher fee, if it's covered at all. Some allow you medications, some don't. The number of days allowed in the hospital must be approved by your insurance. Take the time to understand what's going to be done to you and what's covered, beforehand, unless in an emergency situation where you have no choice as your life is at risk. If you aren't able, then have your caregiver or loved one available to get an understanding for you. Once the procedure is done it's on you, the policyholder, to make sure it's paid. Ignorance of the law, or in this case your policy, is no excuse, legal defense or escape from payment.

As we've discussed, never be afraid or embarrassed to discuss financial issues before you're committed to paying for a procedure, service or test performed on you. I can't stress this enough! You must "actually" read the information and forms you sign before getting your test done. Don't be rushed or pressured to hurry up until you understand what you've read. If you haven't checked or had the staff performing the service get preauthorization for the service, you're committing to paying for the service. Don't assume it's covered. You know what they say about assuming? Do your homework!

There are so many little things to be aware of and the frustration level can be high. Here's something of non-logic to watch out for, although minor, still a good example. When I have lab work done for blood tests they're covered 100%. In other words I pay nothing. But if they check my blood sugar level by poking my finger one time with the exact meter (One Touch) which I use multiple times a day at home, then my insurance policy charges me $12. $12 out of my pocket for doing one time what I do multiple times at home! Needless to say after they got me once we don't perform that test anymore although my doctor orders it every time. I stop the nurse before she pokes my finger and in turn provide a reading of my blood sugar levels for the past month. I'm better off with my process anyway; however, this example shows what the doctor ordered is not always what needs to be done, based strictly on insurance coverage.

Most HMO policies, the type I have, also have pricing structures in which you must use certain doctors (Primary Care Physicians or PCPs) in certain networks (same medical facilities) in order to get the best price. If you go out of the network you'll pay the next level up and so on. This is called the Tier Pricing Structure and is used because the insurance company negotiates pricing for patient referrals within the medical groups. If my endocrinologist orders X-rays I must drive to the medical center miles away to have the X-rays performed instead of using a facility just downstairs from his office in the same building because they aren't in my network. In most cases money drives these decisions instead of practical health care sense or consideration for the patient's transportation costs. There are other policies where you can see any doctor you want at any medical facility (as long as they accept your insurance), but you'll pay a lot higher premium for this luxury.

You must determine which options best suit your needs.

Having proper health care insurance will make a dent in your pocket financially and eat away at your gross pay but not having proper health care insurance can wipe you out financially. A lot of companies are cutting their benefits and putting more of the cost on employees. They cite high health care cost as the main reason why they're in financial trouble, instead of maybe looking at the quality of the product they're selling, or not selling. There are even companies making a profit who are cutting health care benefits for employees and retirees, along with pensions. This is a dangerous trend! If you're in the corporate world please fight for your rights as a worker to get affordable health care coverage and other quality of life benefits. Whether you agree with them or not you must admit the New York Transit union used their power to keep their pensions in early 2006. Desperate times call for desperate measures!

If you're young and think health care will never affect you...wrong! I promise you a time will come when you'll be a patient even though I know you feel nothing will ever happen to you. Think of the future! I felt the same when I was in my 20's and look at me now. Health care is so important to your overall quality of life both now and in your future. Don't take it lightly!

So what do you do when you've done everything right and billing issues arise? Part of learning and understanding your insurance policy beforehand also includes understanding the process to take in case of issues, especially the appeal process. It's important when issues arise you follow these procedures in order to save time and effort on your part because it's probably going to take some time and effort regardless. It's important to understand when you're wasting your time and where to go to get results. Don't waste your time beating your head against a brick wall with someone who has no authority to do anything about your issue and do not let anyone intimidate you into giving in when you know you're right. Usually people will get defensive or use intimidation practices when they have no clue as to what to do, do not want to admit they're wrong or maybe just don't care. Remember my oral surgeon example? Always stand up for your rights!

Most policies have a prewritten process to follow to resolve issues. Issues can arise from something as simple as not having your insurance information updates thus submitting your claim incorrectly, submitting your claim to your supplementary carrier instead of your primary, submitting the wrong form, entering the wrong procedure code or possibly some other incorrect information You don't have to understand all of the ins and outs of how a claim is processed to get results. If you know when you had an appointment or test, what was done during the appointment or why the test was needed and if the appointment or test was covered beforehand, all you need to do is follow the process of the insurance company to get results. It's a good idea to save all of your test results provided by your doctor and if they don't provide you with your results in writing, ask for them. Proper documentation is the key.

Understanding the appeal process and having the proper documentation or notes helped me win every appeal I've had with my insurance company from the oral surgery situation to getting the brand name DDAVP instead of paying the outrageous calculation, or using the generic version that didn't work, to not having to pay for an emergency room visit for my daughter in which nothing was done (I'll explain that one in a second). It's equally important to make your doctor aware of any insurance issues, as their documentation and support could be the deciding factor in winning your appeal. I can't count the number of times my doctors have came through for me in financial related issues due to our positive relationships.

Honest, consistent documentation is a vital key to successfully fighting any billing issues. That's yet another reason why keeping a record of all of your visits, medications and what was discussed in a notebook, or other media, will make it easier to remember to date what took place because sometimes it takes months before the billing issue is reported to you. Without having written the information down you might forget an important detail. Consistency with detail makes fighting any issues run smoother.

Not only is it important to understand how to fight an issue but also when to fight an issue. It's the crying wolf theory all over again when you're always complaining or trying to fight issues that aren't really issues. An issue is when you're not allowed something you're entitled to, are billed for something you didn't receive, or billed for something incorrectly. It doesn't matter how small it might be, at least for me that is, because it's the principle that counts to me. Knowing when to advocate for yourself whether it be billing issues, bad service from a medical professional or correcting any wrong you feel is worth advocating for is everyone's responsibility. If we all fight injustice then maybe justice will prevail and our health care cost will someday be affordable.

Here's the detail of a good example I mentioned briefly earlier. Once I had to spend a couple of nights in the hospital and about a month later I received a detailed Explanation Of Benefits from Medicare stating I had been denied coverage. This was correct because Medicare was my secondary insurance and the hospital had billed them as primary. That issue was easily corrected but as I recommend everyone do, I read the detail and found two things incorrectly billed. I found I had been billed $325 a night for using a CPAP machine (used for sleep apnea) for a total of $650. I had brought my own CPAP machine so I didn't use theirs. Even if I did $325 a night just to use a CPAP machine is a ridiculous profit. I even saw their machine and it was older than mine, which I've had since 2000 and this was 2005. I was also charged $479 for pharmacy use when I had brought my own medications with me when I was rushed to the emergency room and therefore never used the pharmacy. This was a total of $1,129 my insurance company was going to be charged, and incorrectly pay, for services I never received.

My primary policy covers hospital visits 100% so I wasn't going to owe any money for the visit. Therefore these charges weren't any money out of my pocket, or were they? There were two things that bothered me about these charges, aside from $325 a night for use of a CPAP machine was out of this world and could be termed as legal robbery. The first was the hospital and pharmacy was getting paid for services and medications they didn't supply. This, in my opinion, is no different than the corporate CEO stealing from their employees or someone shoplifting from the local market. Of course the shoplifter will get a long jail term and the CEO and medical facility won't do any time, in fact will probably make a healthy profit...but that's another book. The person who submitted the invoice knew I didn't use their CPAP machine nor that they provided me with medications because it was written in my chart. I saw the nurse log it, plus no one ever brought a machine or medications. It's just intentionally wrong! No excuses accepted! If you didn't provide a service then you don't write out a bill for it...period!

Secondly, in reality, it doesn't matter if it's the crooked CEO, raising supply cost or a result of the juvenile shoplifter the employee or consumer pays the price in the end when corporations have to pay out of their profits. Without a doubt if my insurance company pays high fees then eventually "our" premiums will go up. When any business loses money from theft or high prices they always pass on that cost to their customers. That's just how business works and the insurance business is no different. So the reality is even though I might not pay this incorrect bill out of pocket this time, it will affect us sometime in the future. To me it's worth the time and effort to correct it now.

I spent about 45 minutes to an hour calling Medicare, my HMO and the hospital billing department explaining I used my own CPAP machine and medications and these services should not have been billed nor should they be paid. In about a month I got a return courtesy call from the hospital (which I thought was very professional) informing me an audit had been done and I was correct. The charges had been taken off and a new invoice had been sent to my correct insurance company. Even though I never received any thank you from my HMO, which I didn't expect but it would have been a nice customer relations touch, it made me feel good inside to know I had done the right thing and in the end saved patient's money somewhere down the road, even if it did take a little time and effort out of my day. What still bugs me is if they hadn't billed Medicare by mistake I never would have received the detail of the bill and never would have known about the $1,129 incorrect charges because I never receive a detailed Explanation Of Benefits from my HMO for hospital stays. It makes you wonder how often this happens and because of situations like this our premiums rise.

Here's the example I hinted of earlier of not accepting proper medical care and bad customer service. When my daughter was in her early teenage years she was experiencing an extreme sore and swollen throat along with a fever. We took her to the emergency room that evening and as most times, especially before the minimum time wait guarantee you now see in urban emergency rooms, at least in the Detroit area, we had to wait several hours before she was called back to a room. After waiting in the room for quite a while the doctor finally came in. Within no more than three or four minutes and just looking "at" her throat very briefly, he gave her a Motrin and told her she just had a sore throat. He was then on his way before we could even ask him a question.

The next day we went to her PCP and we found out she had an infection. Her PCP was furious about our emergency room visit and didn't understand how anyone who looked "down" her throat couldn't have seen the infection. Hmm, maybe that was the problem as he looked "at" her throat instead of "down" her throat! Her doctor prescribed some medications and in a few days she was okay.

When I got home I called my insurance company and explained the situation and what our PCP had stated. I also provided them my complaint in writing. As a result I was never billed my $50 co-pay for emergency room visits and my insurance company never sent me an Explanation Of Benefits saying they had paid anything as well. Anytime you get unsatisfactory service from any medical service, just like you would with bad service at a restaurant, complain professionally with documentation to back up your complaint and follow the proper channels your insurance company or the medical facility dictates. Don't accept anything unjust to you be it an incorrect bill or bad customer service...ever!

Advocating for yourself is a responsibility we all have. Look at every situation and do what you have to in order to get the proper health care you need. Never be afraid to fight against any wrong. There are always exceptions to the rules. Don't be afraid, as the catch phrase goes, to step out of the box sometimes. Never be afraid to use whatever resources are available to you and take the time to research every option you might have. Just make sure you follow the correct procedures, have all of the required information available and have your doctor or whoever else is involved informed and up to date...then go for it. The worst thing that can happen is you're denied and you're just right back where you started. On the other hand, you never know unless you try. Personally I can live with being told "no", but I could never live with the question "what if?" because I didn't try.

Another movie (also on DVD) I would like to recommend to emphasizes this point, is "John Q". The message of the movie is to show a parent doing what he/she must do in order to get medical treatment when your insurance policy you've paid on for years and years doesn't cover you or your family when you need it. "John Q" is a movie starring Denzel Washington as a father who must get medical attention for his dying son but no one will help him, not his insurance company nor the medical facility. Although it goes to the extreme, and I don't recommend taking it that far, it does give insight on the struggles people have with medical attention and insurance coverage. It's worth your time to check it out because, movie or not, these things do happen.

Aside from your primary insurance coverage, be it any of the options we have discussed, there are other options that need to be considered. First is supplementary insurance, which is a policy that will cover whatever your primary insurance might not cover. For me I currently have an HMO through my wife's employer and Medicare as a supplement. Whatever my HMO doesn't cover, Medicare will, once I've met my deductibles and satisfy their specific calculations regarding the price charged. Of course, whatever is left over after that is my responsibility. In my parents case they have Medicare as a primary then whatever Medicare doesn't cover Aflac, their supplementary carrier, picks up. Supplementary insurance is something you must decide if it's right for your individual health circumstance. This should be thought of during your evaluation of your upcoming health care needs prior to committing to an annual policy. Thinking about supplementary coverage after the fact doesn't do you any good.

When determining if you need a supplementary policy take these questions into consideration. How is your health and do you know of any upcoming situations you need to prepare for such as surgery? Are you willing and able to pay the additional premium, as some supplementary policies are somewhat expensive, even if you never use it? How much is peace of mind worth to you? Is the cost worth the insurance in case you need it? What's not covered under your primary policy? Could you get coverage elsewhere? As you can see a lot of thought needs to go into any decision you make regarding your health care coverage... beforehand! As with your primary policy take the time and effort to research and understand what you need and are getting so you will not be caught in a situation where you can't get the medical attention you need or either your financial future is destroyed. Financial issues are an important and real factor in health care and quality of life. Don't take your financial situation and the consequences lightly.

There are several other options of coverage that might not be covered in your primary policy but are extremely important to your overall health: thus you need to look closely at the detail of your policy to see if you're covered. Dental insurance is the first that comes to mind. As with all medical situations dental care can be quite expensive.

With dental coverage you usually have a different carrier providing this policy. Another important feature usually involved with dental coverage is a yearly limit on the amount you're able to spend, making planning even more important and confusing. We have the premium coverage for dental. However in 2006 I had a restoration (cavity filled) and a crown put on, and then another restoration and root canal all done by January 12th. The total charges billed were $1,991 and my yearly limit is $1,500. As a result I was covered 85% up to $1,500 then the remaining $491 was out of pocket for me. Now even though I've used up my limit and any remaining dental work I have done in 2006 will be 100% out of pocket, except for one cleaning, I still must pay the monthly premium for the remainder of the year. I know of many people who have dental coverage but will not go to the dentist unless they're in unbearable pain because they either don't want to use up their maximum limit or have already used it. I guess you could say they (or me in 2006) have insurance without having insurance. Welcome to the real world!

Another area of importance is vision. Vision is normally included, for a fee, within your primary policy and can be taken outside of your hospital area, such as a vision center in the mall. Your eye sight is something, like your teeth, you only have one set so make sure you keep your eyes checked regularly. Don't be one of those people who won't wear glasses because they think they don't look good. Being able to see is more important than your looks, plus you can look just as cool, intelligent, sexy or whatever other look you want while wearing glasses. Eyewear has now become a fashion statement. I once worked with a man who had so much trouble seeing, because his arms weren't long enough to stretch the distance he needed to get focused, yet he would not wear glasses. He would proudly say, "Now that I'm 40 I refuse to drive a minivan or wear glasses" as if that made him macho or smart. As soon as he would leave the room everyone would comment on how stupid such an intelligent man could be when ego takes over the thinking process. Don't be the blind idiot when your insurance will allow you to wear glasses.

Vision coverage is needed to help with glasses, which without insurance, like everything else medical, can be expensive regardless of the cool ads you see everywhere with cheap designer eyewear. When you're finished you will ask yourself what happen to the ad price? Other vision problems such as seeing an ophthalmologist (a medical doctor who specializes in the eyes) is normally covered under your primary insurance policy since you would see them for problems such as eye diseases or eye surgery. As always look at your individual needs ahead of time to determine what coverage you think will best fit your lifestyle but don't forget your eyes because without them you'll be living in a dark world.

Some other areas of health care insurance to consider are long-term care and life insurance. Long-term care insurance takes care of your needs if you become disabled and can't take care of yourself for a long period of time. Don't confuse long-term care with hospice. Hospice care is when there's nothing else that can be done for a person due to a life ending condition, such as my father with lung cancer. Hospice will take care of all your needs associated with the condition, including medications; however, you can only stay in hospice for a one-year period. Hospice is provided separate from your insurance policy and not something for which you need to pay, as it's normally provided through a medical facility based on documentation from a doctor.

Hospice is a wonderful service provided not only to the patient but to the caregiver as well, even after the patient has passed. My only personal experience with hospice was by way of Big Bend Hospice located in Tallahassee/Perry Florida in association with the care of my father for about nine months. They provided outstanding support covering all medications, supplying home equipment, answering questions at any time, or coming to the house when needed. In addition they gave supportive advice during his illness, provided music therapy when he was in a coma state, and after his death they were there to support my mother in her grief. Big Bend Hospice made a major impact on everyone in our family during the last nine months of my father's life. I don't know what we would have done without them!

Long-term care on the other hand is for when your condition disables you to the point you can't fully take care of yourself but there's no medical reason why you won't live longer than one year. Even if you have an insurance policy, supplementary coverage, receive Social Security or Social Security disability benefits, Medicare or Medicaid, long-term care could still be needed and not covered without a long-term care policy, causing not only stress on your families' lives but financial burdens as well. Old age and conditions associated with aging is one reason for long-term care. Stroke victims are another. There are too many situations to name as reasons for long-term care but it's something everyone should invest in regardless of your current health state. It only takes a split second for an incident to cause you to be disabled for life.

Once that incident happens and you haven't invested in long-term care don't think you will be able to get it after the fact. I've tried for years from independent agents and through my wife's employer to get covered for long-term care but because of my preexisting conditions I'm always denied. If you've heard the rumor you can't be turned down for preexisting conditions take it from me, the reality is, I and many others like me, are turned down on a daily basis. From a business perspective we're a high-risk investment. Take long-term care seriously while you can get it because you never know!

Another thing to consider, before the fact, are policies such as a cancer policy while you're still young and in good health. My father took one out years ago and actually had forgot about it until his agent reminded him of it when he was diagnosed with lung cancer the first time. You can usually have only one policy with a one-time payment of benefits. For my father it was a lifesaver financially. While you're young and in good health is the perfect time to look to your future and anticipated health changes while insurance policies are still available to you at a lower rate. Another good investment for most people (if you can afford it) is a policy to pay off your mortgage if someone in the family dies. I've seen many individuals benefit from this policy when a spouse passed. You can't get around the fact insurance is a real requirement in America. Preparation today will be golden in your future time of need!

Life insurance is another area of health care insurance you want to make sure you have, especially if you have a family. Life insurance is something you should get while you're young and in good health as well, because like long-term care once you develop health conditions, good luck. My wife is able to get some coverage on me via her employer but no one else will provide me with additional funds or policy. Life insurance is critical when death occurs as the average funeral costs in 2006 range from $6,500 to $7,500 for just the basics, and I do mean basics. There are laws that limit the expense funeral homes can charge for specific items so check your state laws now or have someone with a clear head check when it's needed. Being prepared beforehand will ensure your family doesn't endure your death as a burden and can grieve your death in peace.

Speaking of being prepared let me tell you something extremely smart my mother did years back. She purchased everything involved with the funerals for me, my father and herself years ago, paying for it on a payment plan. In fact, she said she wasn't going to retire until she had the funeral arrangements paid for, and she didn't. There's so much involved when a person dies such as getting the casket, vault, grave site, funeral expense, planning the funeral, writing the obituary, distributing property and many other little things. My mother has everything planned and paid for so when the time comes there's nothing the family has to do but grieve. At the time no one wanted to talk about what she was doing and to be honest no one helped her very much, except when she made us mad. Then we would help just to shut her up. However, that didn't stop her and today she has proven how smart she is and how afraid/dumb we were for making it difficult on her! To top it off she got everything at 1980s prices, which for my father saved us approximately $4,700. Smart woman!

You hear some people say, "When I go just split everything up", but it's not that easy. First if no will or trust is written and documented the government is going to take whatever property and decide who gets it. Probate court can hold up the distribution of property for over a year and if an attorney is required, as mandated in certain cities, that will cost the family unnecessary monies, along with any filing costs as well. There's also the cruel reality of family members being at their worst when it comes to getting money or property. You might not think your family will act like that, but that's what many families have said in the past or in court. Like everything regarding insurance and your health, be prepared ahead of time. Funerals are for the living and it's the living who pay the financial burdens. Don't leave that burden on your loved ones! Get prepared while you are still in good health.

Understanding your health care benefits and insurance policies beforehand, no matter how overwhelming and frustrating it may be, will save you money and possible health issues in the end. I'm not going to sugarcoat it, getting a good comfortable understanding of what you're entitled to is tough, overwhelming and frustrating. There will be intimidation not only from the quantity of material and fine print you must soak up but also when you need help, it might be hard to find and a lot of hurdles to jump. Listen closely to what your insurance agent tells you and slow them down so you understand. If they can't explain it to your understanding, get someone who can. You must always remember you, the patient/policyholder, is responsible for the cost of any health care work you have done. Don't be naïve or misinformed. Just because you have insurance doesn't mean you're covered!

…12…

Do all you can to obtain and maintain health care insurance. It is a must in our current health care environment and to your future, regardless of your current health condition. Always remember this about health care – health don't care! Think about it!!!

14
To Be Honest Or Be Silent

I've stressed the importance of honesty throughout this book and given example after example of how honesty is the only way to build successful relationships – get the proper understanding between individuals – relay how you feel healthwise and emotionally to your medical professionals and caregivers in order to get the positive help you need – make it through legal processes – fight wrongful bills – get financial assistance – ensure your children understand, honesty allows you to better cope with your health situation – and most importantly, enables you to accept and deal with your life from a personal perspective. From a moral standpoint honesty is something, regardless of how hard it might be at times, we all must practice, even more so for those in public service. In fact you're probably sick of me mentioning it, but hopefully the philosophy is now imbedded in your brain, as I throw a twist to the equation. There's one area in our society where honesty, in my opinion, is still the only way to go, but unless we have some major changes in culture, honesty is not going to be a priority, especially in regard to health. I'm talking about the employee to employer relationship in corporate America!

Most people will do whatever they must in order to get a better job to support themselves and their families financially, including not being honest. The thing is it always catches up to you, if not immediately, eventually. You can get the job by saying you have vast experience using a word processor, but as soon as you sit down alone to produce your first document the truth will be in the writing. In order to get the job you want at the local car dealership you can testify how you've been repairing cars since you were in high school but as soon as your first blown transmission rolls up on your rack, you're in need of a tow truck. You can proclaim yourself the greatest chef on the planet having created many popular recipes but as soon as a hungry customer tastes your first meal the truth is out and you're burnt toast. It doesn't matter how deep you look into your interviewers' eyes and praise yourself about all of the monies you saved your previous company during your last job as a financial analyst, as soon as the results from your lack of knowledge or experience for making sound financial decisions from your last job as a cashier costs your new company a large sum of money your scam is revealed.

Some people can hustle better than others and get away with it to become successful, for a while. When I worked in the corporate world I once knew a man who had been with the company for years and couldn't read. He would have his wife write his memos from memory or work in a group but never was the one to take notes or put out the final document, just provide input to the process. Finally, my manager caught him as he put him on the spot by asking him to simply write the minutes from a meeting, in the next 30 minutes. There was no one in the office at the time to help him or proof his work and when my manager saw the result he knew something wasn't right. I'm not sure whatever happened to him but his situation isn't unique. Just like I learned to hide my health condition for years he learned the same tricks regarding his reading ability. The thing is at the end of the day honesty always comes to the forefront. Your health situation is no exception!

I think I've gotten more looks as to say, "Gil, you're absolutely crazy!" when I make this statement than any other statement I've made, and I've actually made some crazy statements in my lifetime; but here goes, "You've got to be honest and upfront about your health condition and how it will affect your ability to be a productive employee with your employer." Okay you can stop the crazy look and let me explain!

The employee/employer relationship is no different from any other relationship. You're a team with the same primary objective, both parties being successful in what they do, which in turn makes the business successful. That's the bottom line and in business it's all about the bottom line!

Another bottom line is if you have a chronic health condition or someone at home has a health situation in which you're a primary caregiver the time will come when it affects your job. As was my case, you aren't able to make it physically, without warning, to the office on certain days, or you have to go to a number of doctor appointments or treatments, take medications that have predictable and unpredictable side effects, or must at times leave the job to care for a chronically ill patient. You owe it to your employer and to yourself to be upfront about your situation. The truth is if your employer can't handle the situation upfront then not being honest with him/her might get you the position but when the time comes, and it will come, when you need support, what then?

I understand reality and why people sometimes are dishonest in interviews regarding their health situation. They might feel it's no one's business and has nothing to do with them doing the job plus they legally don't have to talk about it. The applicant may feel the employer won't look at his/her work skills and how valuable he/she could be to the business but instead shy away as a result of a health situation, which I must admit is probably true the majority of the time. However if your health affects your ability to perform on a regular basis without some understanding and minor adjustments, then it does impact your ability to do the job. It doesn't mean you wouldn't be successful and the best person for the job, it just means both you and your employer need to be on the same page.

I understand the need to survive as well, as Mother Nature looks after us all. If you're in need to get employment in order to support yourself or your family and you're at the end of your rope then Mother Nature's instinct for survival will take over and you'll say whatever is needed in order to get the job. Desperate times call for desperate measures and understandably so, especially in the times we live in today where even those with skills, master degrees and morality or virtue have done the right thing all their lives are unemployed. The fact still exists your health situation remains the same regardless of what job you apply for or what you say in an interview. We all do what we have to do to survive and life puts us in certain situations where we have to make tough decisions. I just hope honesty will always be your primary choice.

As an employer you can make it easier for the employee to be honest from the start. When you're describing the position and your organization make it clear you support health and family issues fully, as long as the requirements of the job are met. After all this is business. Let the future employee know upfront if they have special circumstances then adjustments will be made and resources will be provided for them to fulfill their responsibilities, but you must know beforehand of these needs in order to provide the resources, not after deadlines are about to be missed. It's up to the employer, both for future and current employees, to set the corporate culture so honesty is not punished but rewarded. In the end not only will the business relationship be successful but the bottom line will be successful as well. Isn't that the real objective in any business?

With that said…if an employee is upfront about his/her health situation then one of two things will take place. The first is you won't get the job or the employer will put such demands and requirements on the position you won't accept it. The truth is, in this case, although illegal and their actions should be reported, this employer isn't worth working for to begin with. Find another opportunity! If you take the job you're going to have problems in the future when you need their support. You could tell yourself if you become a valuable employee when the time for support comes your employer will see your value and have a change of heart. Maybe, but I wouldn't bet a career on it. Your best bet, like with any red flag, is to walk away, if at all possible. Again I understand desperate times require desperate measures and sacrifice. The bottom line problem is the employee, the employer and the business suffers unnecessarily in the end.

The second option, and the one that should take place, based on the fact your job skills meet the job requirements, is to see if the two of you can come to a compromise that will not only benefit you both, but more importantly, benefit the business. Not only is it the law, based on the Americans With Disability Act (ADA), but it's good business practice as well. The ADA, or Public Law 101-336, is a federal law enacted on July 26, 1990 that prohibits discrimination and ensures equal opportunity for persons with disabilities in employment. Just because you have a disability or chronic health condition doesn't mean you can't be the top performer in an occupation. This is especially true for individuals who might have already been employed for a number of years before their health deteriorates.

It's a lot more cost efficient for a business to make adjustments to obtain a productive employee than to go out and hire someone new, although in most cases the new employee will be paid a lot less. Not only does the employer have the required training time and therefore a drop in productivity, it's just the right thing to do and will benefit the morale status of your employees. Never underestimate the impact of morale in a business!

In my case when I was diagnosed with sarcoidosis I got out of management and into a Business Analyst position to better utilize my skill sets and allow me to be able to not be physically in the office at all times and still meet my requirements. In addition I'm extremely organized so if I wasn't there and someone needed information they could always look on my desk and find exactly what they wanted. I carried a pager (this was the 1990s) and constantly checked my voice mails, unless I was unable due to an emergency situation. I was honest with my management, co-workers, and customers about my health situation. Because they understood I was available when not in the office, they didn't feel they were disturbing me. I updated my voicemail's outgoing message on a regular basis so anyone would know if I was physically in the office or not, therefore my co-workers, management, or customer would have an idea when I would be returning their call, along with leaving an emergency contact if immediate action was needed. In addition they could always send me an e-mail that I could check from home. These were adjustments I made to ensure my responsibilities were met, and as a result they were.

Now even though I met my requirements and had no complaints from my management, co-workers, and customers, at least to me that is, I'm sure there must have been some behind my back. I know deep down inside it would have been easier for everyone involved if I had been able to be in the office on a daily basis, which is why I'm sure there were comments when I wasn't around…people will always be people in the office environment. Some co-workers who didn't know the details of how I checked voicemails when I wasn't in the office, worked from home or knew the extent of my health issues (after all I didn't look sick and rumors are always present in the office environment) might have thought it wasn't fair or maybe I got special treatment. That's just something that's always going to be present in the workplace and always has been so allowing a productive employee adjustments to ensure he/she can still remain productive is not going to change human nature. Instead concentrate and judge each employee based on his/her performance and ensure clear-cut processes and feedback is in place so the results and reasons are as clear as spring water. Holding everyone accountable, regardless of his/her personal situation, will allow the bottom line to continue to be successful and that's what really matters from a business standpoint, as the bottom line only cares about the bottom line.

In the business world the relationship between employee and employer is a two way street and no one owes the other anything. Instead you owe each other everything. Success in business is a team effort. There's no room for self-pity or feeling the other owes you something for nothing. As an employer you pay your employees to do a job and you expect them to perform as required. However the employer owes the employee the resources and support, physical, financial and emotional, to be able to meet those requirements. As the employee you're paid to do a job and meet the requirements you agreed to meet when you took the position. You owe your employer the honest effort to do everything in your power to meet those requirements.

Business is a give and take relationship. If an employee is allowed to take off work during regular business hours, for personal or health related reasons, it shouldn't be a big deal if the employee comes in outside of regular business hours or works from home to ensure their responsibilities are met. You owe that respect to your employer. If an employee meets their requirements and goes beyond just showing up for work then going home or having a need to take care of health related situations, during "normal" business hours, shouldn't be a problem with the employer. You owe that respect to your employee. Together and on the same page is what makes businesses successful. Loyalty is a two way street and until both the employer and the employee change the mindset of it's all about me, which seems to be the mindset of 21st century corporate America and American workers, businesses will suffer and honesty will be the second language.

The business culture must change and I think it starts with corporate America. I totally understand corporations are in business to make a profit and have every right to spread the wealth to whomever they choose. That's the American way. If you don't like it start your own business. It just seems to my simple logical mind in order for successful businesses to be profitable and be fair, the profits should be spread around or at the least make it down to the employees who actually do the majority of the work to support the core of the business? Don't people put more loyalty and effort into something they profit from or could possibly lose from as well based on their performance? Wouldn't the business profit more if everyone felt the results, both profit and losses, instead of executives making millions regardless while the actually workers get their benefits, pensions, salaries and jobs cut even when the business profits? Maybe it's just me but there's something wrong with that picture! I think by now (especially now) we have proven the "Trickle Down" theory (the belief if you make the rich richer they'll pass their wealth to others in less fortunate situations thus we all profit) doesn't work. No the rich just keep the money resulting in the growing divide between the haves and the have-nots.

I've been in management (not at the executive level but I did manage several data centers with numerous employees) and I've been on the front lines. I understand the importance of management's decisions, especially in regard to financial responsibilities, but let's look at reality for a second. I don't care how cost efficient a medical center is run or what management processes are in place if you don't have qualified nurses and doctors, along with other productive staff branches such as lab technicians, transport support, cleaning staff, etc., the medical center is not going to be successful. The same holds true with other businesses as well. An airline can be reduced by management to a lean mean cost efficient operation but if they don't have qualified pilots, courteous customer service staff to assist customers on flights and make the reservations, baggage handlers, mechanics, cleaning staff and the other employees who deal directly with the customers then the airline will not succeed. You can have the best management team in regard to the automobile industry but if you don't have the creative engineers, hard working plant workers to build the cars correctly as well as the support of the car salespeople who deal directly with the public then you'll be blaming health care as to why your cars won't sell.

Why is it the executives get big time bonuses and stock options while the workers get pay cuts, benefits cut, pensions reduced or terminated? "They" say they need to pay executives outrageous amounts to keep a management team to run the business successfully but isn't it the workers who really run the business? I don't see any executives flying any planes, performing any surgeries, keeping the business physically clean and presentable to the customers or providing direct customer service! Until we adjust to a new business culture where everyone is treated fairly, then employers shouldn't expect employees to have honesty as a top priority when health needs are the issue. Is it any surprise employees jump from corporation to corporation depending on which way the wind blows? If you aren't honest with someone or rewarded honesty, why should you expect an employee to be honest with you?

Honesty also needs to be looked at closely when the employee gets to a point where the requirements of the job aren't being met. This is a difficult thing to do for both the employee and employer. From an employee with a chronic health condition's standpoint you already have the tough daily task of looking in the mirror and determining if you can continue to be employed in the same position, or employed at all. For me this was a long process to come to grips with. Family and doctors had told me I shouldn't be working the corporate job I maintained, or partially maintained, for years before I actually left the corporate world. Then it was forced. It wasn't just the cut in pay but the feeling of usefulness I was afraid I would lose that scared me the most. My endocrinologist once told me, although he didn't feel this would happen to me because of my writing and mindset, his biggest concern about people on disability is after a while they stop living life and start living disabled. I didn't want this to happen to me!

Eventually I couldn't function anymore and my inability to perform my job responsibilities started to become noticeable, as I finally honestly accepted my reality. I must say EDS supported me 100% throughout the years, although I gave them 100% as well from both an honesty and effort standpoint. Towards the end my job responsibilities were decreasing and I still had trouble fulfilling my requirements. I was able to work from home and I still met the majority of my requirements without help from co-workers but the toll on my health was obvious. So finally the decision was made to include me in a staff reduction and I left the corporate world, with mutual respect, in April 2002 (11 years after my official diagnosis of sarcoidosis). Business is business, regardless if you have or manage someone with a chronic health condition, and in some situations reality can be cold! However, it is what it is and must be addressed without prejudice, regardless of the outcome. As life is ever changing so is your career so don't look at the fact you can't work a "regular" job anymore as a negative but instead look at it as a new opportunity to do something else. Life goes on with or without you!

I pray that corporate America will wake up and start providing employees with the culture to promote honesty and reward those who are loyal to their employer while at the same time employees will take pride once again in their jobs. It's going to take both sides coming together to accomplish this goal and in the end corporate America, American workers and consumers worldwide will benefit.

Honesty is questioned in another area in which a decision must be made by the patient as to what information they should give out for their own good. That area is the people outside your inner circle with whom you're associated. Some people love to tell everyone they can how bad they have it healthwise, crying wolf theory again. Most people care about a person's personal life but too much information is not needed nor wanted. It can be a real turn off! Others feel their health is their own business and no one needs to know what they deal with on a personal level. All that's well and dandy but, for your own good, it's necessary to be honest about your health to a degree. It's the degree you must determine. Here's what I mean.

We all care, regardless of what someone might say, to a certain extent, about how other people perceive us. I don't want anyone to feel sorry for me or look at me with pity. In the same tone, from a selfish standpoint, people around me need to have some knowledge of my health condition. At the least they need to know I have chronic health conditions as a result of sarcoidosis and I carry a medical alert card with me that contains in detail my health status in my wallet. The importance of this information is not so they can get to know me in a more personal way or develop some type of bond with them but instead if something happens to me, and with my health condition something could happen at anytime, I want whoever is with me to at least know to react and have some knowledge as to what to tell the EMS folks when they arrive – if nothing but that I have a medical condition and medical alert card in my wallet.

You don't have to give out too much information or information with whom you're uncomfortable because your health situation is strictly your business. Unfortunately some people will shy away from you if they feel you have a health condition – especially one they don't understand. Some people will start showing pity for you as if you can't do anything for yourself anymore even though you were doing fine before you told them of your conditions. As someone with a chronic health condition and legally classified as disabled I can say from personal experience people in similar situations like myself don't want special treatment. I can't think of anything that shows ignorance more than people who will say things like "It must be nice to be off work" when someone is out on a disability leave. I can remember so clearly after I was released from the hospital in 1991 from getting adjusted to my medications and my arms were still aching and bruised (I looked like a heroin addict) from having been injected for five straight days and drained from all of the adjustments, I went to get lunch at a restaurant I frequented on a regular basis. My waitress, who I'd known for years, came up to me and asked me where I had been lately. I told her the truth, as she already knew I had been very sick, and then she asked if I was at lunch break from work. I told her, "No, I just got out of the hospital and won't be going back to work until my doctors clear me" as I wondered if she had heard anything I just said. She looked at me and sincerely commented, "Oh, it must be nice!"

This is why I use the term "ignorance" because let me set the record straight for anyone who says things that inconsiderate, especially if the person actually believes it and not just saying something because he/she has nothing else to say. When someone is talking about health issues some people start getting uncomfortable. There's nothing nice about being sick! If anyone thinks it's nice to be off work because you're sick, require strict bed rest or disabled, please think back to a time when you were sick. Did you enjoy it? Did you have a good time?

You don't make any money to amount to anything, especially compared to the real world. It's not fun to be home on disability and unable to live the normal life you once enjoyed. Trust me and I think I can speak for 95% of people who deal with chronic health conditions or are disabled when I say we would give anything not to be in the position we're in not being able to live our normal lives. Although you can live a positive quality of life on disability if we, or at least I, had the choice to return to our pre-disability life it would be a no-brainer. Please think before you speak! I understand you probably just don't have anything else to say and if that's the case, just smile. You'll make us feel a lot better than your conversation.

The pure reality is we just want to be normal. True we have to make certain adjustments in our life in order to be as normal as we can but we don't want others to treat us any differently or hold us to a lesser standard than anyone else. Instead show us understanding and treat us as you would want to be treated yourself. The results of the attitudes of people, (maybe its human nature, fear or ignorance, toward others not quite like themselves) cause honesty to take a back seat again. As an individual we must determine to whom we provide health information and how much we tell. We can't change human nature and people will be people, but my thing is I want everyone with whom I'm associated to react if I need help! If people want to shy away from me then so be it. I'd rather they shy away than have no idea what to do if I need help. One might cause me not to be friends with someone who I shouldn't be friends with anyway and the other might cost me my life. For me, that's not a difficult choice to make.

Personally anyone from a co-worker to someone I spend time with on a casual basis needs to understand, if I need help as a result of my health reality, how to help me. All I ask is you know to call 911 and tell them I have medical information in my wallet. If they can't deal with the truth or can't handle those two simple tasks – if needed, they don't need to be around me. Honesty is a hard thing to accept at times and dishonesty can make life easier in the short term, but in the end, especially as a patient with chronic health conditions, the truth will come out, whether you're on the job or at a friend's party. For your own sake as a patient, make sure honesty works for you and don't let dishonesty or trying to fit in by hiding your reality cost you your life!

...14...

Honesty is something you should always practice in order to have a successful and fulfilling life as a patient, caregiver, employee, employer, and friend. Your word is what others will judge you on throughout your life. Remember, only you can cause your word to go bad!

15
Sexuality, Diet, And Self-Esteem

Throughout this book we have discussed many aspects of our lives from the importance of faith, relationships, financial awareness, honesty, and accepting changes; to name a few. There are just a few more aspects of life I want to touch on which are affected by our health I feel need to be brought to the forefront, as they can affect your life in a multitude of ways. The first is sexuality. Sexuality!!! I bet I have your attention now? Don't worry it's not XXX rated, just reality rated.

When you look at powerful emotions that can cause a person to do things they later ask themselves, "What the hell did I just do?" sex has to rank at the top of the list, along with financial situations. Sex has caused great men and women, to fall from grace and power – caused individuals to make financial decisions they regretted for years to come – broke up marriages – caused embarrassment for family – caused unwanted children to be brought into this world – spread disease when performed unsafely or as a result of dishonesty when individuals don't inform their partners they have a sexual transmitted disease (in my opinion these people should get life in prison without parole) – caused guilt – and been used as a weapon in the form of rape, both in the free world and in prisons. However, sex can also be a positive act of emotion when used between two people in love, as a form of expressing their love for each other. Other qualifying results of sex are reproduction of life, as a result of family planning – the best makeup to any fight or argument you might ever have (in fact some couples fake arguments just for the makeup sex) – as an outlet to reduce stressful situations in your life – and a multitude of other positive rewarding reasons as well. In addition and probably the most powerful reason thus far, it feels so good!

Although sex should never be the primary reason for a relationship and shouldn't be the most important thing two people have together (in regard to serious relationships), sex is still an important part of a spousal relationship. When health changes such as chronic health conditions, diabetes, aging or other stressful events enter a person's life one of the main things affected is his/her sex life. Issues with your sex life, in turn, affect your relationship and your self-esteem, be you a man or woman.

Some stressful issues such as losing your job, a death in the family, taking care of a loved one or a major decision that needs to be made are some things that could cause you not to perform, or want to perform, sexually. There are ever-present financial issues as well that seem to have an impact on all aspects of your life, including a person's sexuality. Naturally the aging process too is a factor. Menopause is something that can have a negative impact on a sexual activity and affects both parties. It's not just the partner with an issue who is affected since it takes two to tango. The other partner must find a way to deal with the lack of sexual affection as well, which most times, like being a caregiver, is the most difficult to handle.

What's the best way to deal with these sexual issues in a relationship or make your sex life more rewarding when you both aren't functioning at full force? You guessed it…honest communications as to what turns you on. You must understand sexuality is a lot more than just intercourse. It's not only about pleasing yourself but ensuring your partner is pleased as much, if not more, than you. That in itself is self-rewarding, both to the male ego and a woman's romantic emotion.

From the perspective of how a patient's health issues affects his/her sexuality, the individual and the relationship, the real question is what adjustments can be made to get your sex life back to normal? For men, especially younger men under 40, having sexual issues, which may include having problems getting erections, having a decreased desire to perform sex, not having the energy to perform sexually or having premature ejaculation issues, can be devastating to the male self-esteem. These issues will cause depression and a lashing out in other areas, as the stupid male ego wants to prove, "I'm still a man!" Let me set one thing straight to the stupid male ego and anyone who listens to it. Your sexual performances have nothing to do with you being a man! Being a man means taking care of your responsibilities as a man, not how long you can perform sexual intercourse.

The real problem for men is they don't understand why they're having these issues and how simple it could be to get them back to normal.

Most men won't go to their doctor to find out why they're having problems until after they have suffered too long or caused negative impacts on their relationship or to themselves from a mental standpoint! The male upbringing leads him to believe the locker room mentality where a "real" man can perform sex at the drop of a hat for hours on end and at the end of the night the only person who matters is him because all women love him. That's the stupidest logic the male ego has ever come up with, and believe me, all men have been exposed to it and fell for the logic at some point in our lives.

Most men have very few outlets for which they feel comfortable talking about their sexual problems, as they fear being seen as inferior from a man's perspective. Some of us are blessed to have a partner who understands and is supportive, but a lot of us have women who immediately blame themselves, or worse yet put us down, which brings the negative male ego into play, causing additional unnecessary stress on the relationship. Nothing positive ever comes from listening to the stupidity our male egos sometimes teach us! Don't even mention discussing his sexual issues with the fellows. We've already laid out the male ego mentality and the last thing you want is for your male friends to think you're less than a "real" man. I don't care if you're straight, bi or gay, that's one thing all men have in common from a sexual standpoint, our male ego needs to be stroked when it comes to being able to perform sexually. A man can't fake it, we're either up or we're not! We don't fake orgasms either. You know if a man climaxed because it's there for the eye to see. Like most things in a man's makeup, it's I did or I didn't and if I can't my manhood is suspect. Why do you think we love sports so much? You either win or you lose. There's no in between. It doesn't have to be like that.

If you aren't fortunate enough to be able to honestly communicate your feelings with your spouse (a relationship issue in itself) or a close friend you must be able to communicate your issues to the one person who can help – your doctor. Having sexual issues, in most cases, are a result of a medical condition that can be corrected. We aren't embarrassed if we have some other type of health condition that medication can help us get back to normal so why are we so embarrassed about talking to our doctor about sexual issues? I'm not one to blame society but in this case it might be appropriate. Men are trained not to show emotion to begin with and be able to suck up any type of health situation. That's one reason why a man won't go to the doctor unless something is really bothering him and it just won't go away on its own. I must admit I fit into this category at times as you've heard me mention my need to stay strong and be the strong male figure when deaths occur, which I know deep down causes me emotional damage as I hold my emotions inside. The male ego and mentality is a powerful combination, sometimes in a negative way!

Another reason we won't talk to our doctors about health issues as freely as women and something we as men can't admit, is in reality we're afraid of what might be wrong with us when it comes to health issues. We think we're invincible and nothing bad will ever happen to us from a health standpoint. We're taught men are strong and should be able to endure pain at any cost. I call it the "John Wayne mentality". The reality is this logic only causes us to deteriorate healthwise and become worse off than if we had just gone to our doctor for a routine physical or reported everything bothering us when we did go. Women aren't totally excluded from this example either, but men seem to fall for it the majority of the time.

In most cases simple medication, be it for diabetes, hypertension or Erectile Dysfunction (ED), can be taken to correct the source issue causing our sexual issues. The bottom line is you have a medical problem so don't be embarrassed, fix it. Trust me, there are a lot of men, more than you might imagine and some with an extreme macho reputation, who experience sexual issues. You're not alone so don't allow embarrassment or your male ego to make you alone. Adjust your mentality and talk to your partner about how you feel. More importantly, talk to your doctor about your issue and if you can't find it in yourself to be able to talk honestly with your doctor or partner, you need to look at the relationships because something isn't right other than your sexual issues.

A sexual issue isn't just a man's thing! Fellows, believe it or not, women enjoy sex and feel it's an important part of their lives, the same as men. Like we need to forget the locker room mentality we need to forget the Father Knows Best mentality as well because it's not the 1950's anymore. Although a woman's sexual issues aren't as obvious as a man's, societiy's perception is unfairly different as a man who enjoys sex might be labeled positively as a playboy while a woman with the same lifestyle is labeled negatively as a whore. They still exist and are still as damaging to a woman's life as any male sexual issue can be to a man's life.

As a man I've dealt with women at "that time of the month" all my sexually active life and it can be a pain in the butt, to say the least. In fact I experience what my doctor terms "Male PMS" as a result of my insufficient testosterone levels. I get an injection at which time my testosterone levels are high. As the two-week period progresses each day my testosterone levels go down just a little bit until another injection boost them back up again. Therefore every day my hormone levels are different with the mood swings and the whole nine yards, which is "basically" what PMS is all about. I'm not implying I understand what women go through, I'm simply stating I have a better idea since sarcoidosis changed my life.

Hormone adjustments are a common cause for women to experience sexual issues. During and after menopause can cause a woman not to be in the mood as frequently, if at all, or as intense. There are medications and suggestions your medical professional can provide you to help with these issues, but, of course, you must first talk to them, something women will do more frequently and honestly than men (and some say women are the weaker sex and men are the smarter – you decide!).

As a sarcoidosis patient and a patient on prednisone I have talked to many female patients who, as a result of the same sources, too experience sexual issues. As I've said, sex is a lot more than just intercourse. For a woman this is a fact they hold deeper because they have a stronger desire for romance while most men would be satisfied with just sex and then go back to whatever we were doing. Romance, the ability to look sexy for your partner and pleasing your partner are probably more important to a woman than a man, although some of us men folk have those objectives as well.

Don't get me wrong…I'm not trying to promote the sexual stereotype mentalities; I'm trying to break them! My point is having a positive self-esteem is important for achieving positive sexuality. Prednisone, and other drugs, can negatively impact that requirement. Prednisone is a mean drug and is used for so many things we would be here all night listing them. One thing it's obviously used for is treating sarcoidosis. Side effects, although too many to mention again, include immediate weight gain and a puffy face, known as round face. In addition, as I've told you I experienced, it will give you the munchies more than if you had just smoked an ounce of weed (for those of you who know about that kind of thing!), thereby increasing the weight gain even more.

The sudden gain of weight will cause a woman not to feel like herself and certainly not as sexy as she did in the past. Even if her partner tells her sincerely how beautiful she is, unless she can see the beauty in the mirror the compliments fall on deaf ears. Adding to the mix prednisone causes mood swings, well let's just say even the strongest of relationships are in for a test. You can't love someone else until you love yourself, an old cliché but one that's oh so true, especially when making love is involved, which is what sex should be all about. Sometimes it's the mental aspect that's worse to accept than the physical.

Another example of the lack of feeling sexy are people who must use special medical equipment or have special medical needs such as oxygen. I want to you to read an actual excerpt from an e-mail I received from a female sarcoidosis patient to emphasis my point and how facing your situation with understanding heals all.

... "I welcomed the open and honesty of your book as it pertains to sexual dysfunction. Sexual dysfunction as a result of medication, chronic illness, etc. is a subject I wish we could be more open about. Thanks for opening the door to that very real problem that needs discussing. Sexual activity is very strenuous and I thought I would stop breathing if I had intercourse with my husband. So instead I tried to avoid it. He became frustrated and then I became frustrated. Plus I felt unattractive with having a cannoli up my nose giving me oxygen during intimacy. How attractive is that? I overcame it by going deep within my soul and asked, "Do you want to look attractive during intercourse or do you want to be able to breathe and enjoy yourself?" Well, the latter won! The first time my husband asked, "Do you want me to get your oxygen?" before one of our intimate moments I knew that we'd reached a higher level of acceptance, love and understanding. Right today he doesn't know how unattractive I felt with that tube up my nose during intimate moments...or maybe he does. But now it's no big deal and what a difference it made in our lives once we were able to accept my situation as it is. There are a lot of people dying to talk about this but are too embarrassed.*

Thanks for sharing that most private part of your life"...

To me that say's in all! Adjusting to any sexual issue with honesty and understanding will enable you to overcome the obstacle and get back to a normal life, be you a man or woman. I'm not a love doctor but...making love is what it says, expressing physical love with your romantic partner. Don't get hung up on the proper way to express yourself sexually because there is no proper way to express yourself except in the manner that satisfies the two of you. "To each his own." That never had more of a direct reflection on anything than sexual relations. Sex is a fact of life, deal with any issues as such, especially health related ones...without embarrassment!

Another aspect of life that is a primary cause for a multitude of additional physical and mental health issues, regardless of our sex, age or health status is our diet. Our diet is something we all need to adjust to throughout our lives. We are what we eat and there isn't much in our lives that has such an impact on our overall health as our diet, something I think, unless you're in denial, we can all agree on. Why do we have such problems controlling our urge to eat and adjusting to necessary diet changes, to not only improve our health, but at times save our life? When I was going through my symptoms there were two things I had problems with that today I appreciate every single time I do either - make love to my wife and eat! Making love doesn't do me any harm. My diet on the other hand is another story!

I love to eat! Unfortunately, like millions of others, eating doesn't always love me back. I could give you some good excuses like the one about how much I appreciate being able to eat again after not being able to during all those years, or how about I take prednisone daily and that gives me the munchies, or maybe I could blame my wife since she is a wonderful cook and I feel obligated to take advantage of that skill. However, I think the real reason is my lifetime love to eat out. I could go on with more excuses but you get the picture, plus I'm sure most of you could come up with a few better ones for me to use as well.

Everyone has his/her weaknesses when it comes to diet. Mine is cheeseburgers! I love them and eat them on a regular basis. Fast food, homemade, on the grill, at a sit down restaurant, ground beef or turkey burger, it doesn't matter, I can't get enough. Of course I know too many cheeseburgers causes me health issues I could prevent if I would limit my consumption but that's the thing with eating. For most of us it's so damn hard to control!

Adjusting to a proper diet, whether you're healthy or not, can eat anything or have special diet needs, young or old, rich or poor, hungry or got the munchies, is one of the hardest things in life to do, and even more so, stick with on a regular basis. The thing is, a proper diet is one of the most important aspects of anyone's life in regard to maintaining good health and even more important in managing any health condition.

The foods we consume is the fuel that makes our bodies function. I bet if we knew the real truth, which we never will, the majority of health conditions could be traced back to, and either prevented or lessened, as a result of our diet. When we're healthy we don't think about all of the sugar and junk food we eat but in the end diabetes, dental issues and a number of other health problems come our way. Properly managing our diet, and our children's diets as well, is our personal responsibility and the results can't be changed once your food choices have entered your body. Talk about the need for will power! Diet is the number one challenger in the will power battle, at least for most of us. For those individuals who win, the will power verse diet war, you have my ultimate respect!!!

So what should you eat to maintain proper health? To whom should you listen? Those are two hard questions! Let me start with number two. I don't know to whom to listen to because what you're supposed to eat and what you aren't changes on a weekly basis. I go back to the question regarding results of any study. Who funded it and who will benefit the most from the findings? If the cattle industry is involved in a study on how red meat affects individuals the results will show red meat does you no harm and actually does you good. The poultry industry will then come out with a study showing how red meat harms you and chicken is the way to go. Of course after them the fishing industry will come out with something showing how seafood is the ultimate health meat to consume. When it comes to helping reduce a specific disease the wine industry will come out with study results showing a glass of wine a day does wonders. Not to be outdone, the citrus growers will let you know, based on their studies, fruit is nature's diet sensation. One thing I can tell you for sure…if any of the studies in the above examples had any negative results, you wouldn't hear about them! That's all I can guarantee you or be sure of! Something else to think about – ever wonder why there are so many different diets and books to instruct you how to lose weight, making a ton of monies I might add, based on the studies of the food industry? Then they go away…

For me there are three resources for you to listen to in regard to your diet. First is your doctor. Your doctor knows your specific health needs and what foods would benefit you. Of course, make sure they aren't associated with any special hot diet products or getting any kick-backs from recommending a specific diet. But then you already trust your doctor's advice based on the positive relationship you have together – right? If referred by your doctor, a dietician is another good resource but use one your doctor recommends and not a popular one trying to promote a book or specific diet. Not that diet books are bad it's just you want your health needs to be the top priority and not a secondary agenda for your adviser.

The second, and maybe most important resource, listen to your body. We've already established your body will give you warnings if something isn't right for you. Having heartburn from spicy food is a warning for you not to eat spicy food. Feeling miserable after eating certain foods or too much food in general is your body giving you warning signs you need to adjust to what you just gave your body or your body is going to make your life miserable or just stop functioning. Listen to what your body tells you and adjust because once your body has used up the warnings you're stuck with the results for life, which brings me to the third resource – common sense.

Common sense is something we seem to lack from time to time, especially when our diet is concerned. However, it's a trait to which every individual should listen to regarding not only your diet, but your other life situations as well, including your overall health, as common sense is just another way your inner voice speaks to you. You know when it comes to the answer to the first question of what should we eat, common sense seems to be the perfect solution.

Let me say once again I'm only a patient. I'm not a doctor or dietician, have no connections to specific diets, don't really control my own diet very well, never conducted or participated in any diet related studies and most of all I love to eat. With that said, diets come and go, allowing individuals and corporations to make millions off of people desperate to control their diets or look like falsely beautiful people they see in magazines. Then the next study, funded by another diet or food group who was excluded in the hot diet, will conclude the logic behind the hot diet is false and now this diet (which happens to include their food group) is the only way to go. Bam…another individual and corporation makes millions while the consumer is so confused they just eat whatever they want in the end anyway and never stick with either popular by the minute diet.

Here's the personal opinionated Gilbert Barr's diet suggestion. Eat a variety of food groups as long as your body doesn't give you any warning signs that you have a specific health condition. As an example, if you're diabetic stay away from foods that cause your sugar levels to rise, whatever they may be. Don't concentrate on a specific food but instead get all of the food groups in your body because they all, or at least most, help at least one area of your body. Last, and most important, control your portions of all your food consumption.

Portions are the real key to any diet and personally my biggest problem to control. Eating the proper portions of a variety of food groups gives your body the proper balance and nutrition without overdoing it.

Another important adjustment you must make, and Lord knows I wish I was better at this, is don't eat if you aren't hungry. Might sound logical but how many times have you finished your plate when you could have stopped half way through and saved the rest for later? How many times have you had "that" desert when you were already stuffed but it just looks so good, plus it's right there and you don't want it to go to waste or someone else eat it? How many times have you, out of pure habit, grabbed a snack to watch the game even though you just had dinner or it was the time of night when you automatically grab a snack while you're watching television? How many times has someone told you or you told yourself, "My eyes were bigger than my stomach" but since you have it you don't want to waste it so you eat it? After all haven't we all been told since a kid when we don't eat all of our food, "Do you know how many starving people there are in the world that would kill to have your food? Don't you waste it!" So what do we do? We become a member of the clean plate club, a club most of us don't need to belong! We've done them all and, in turn, paid for them all in the long run!

One of the best ways to curb your cravings to eat and at the same time help you stay healthy is to drink as much water as you can. Personally I hate plain water, but that's just my downfall. It has no taste and I would much rather have a Diet Pepsi (I've learned to drink caffeine-free which has improved my ability to get a better night's sleep), lemonade or ice tea. Over time I've learned to add real lemon to my water if I need taste, which works for me. I've also started taking a bottle of water to bed with me instead of a soft drink. I've even learned to grab a cold bottle of plain water when I just need a quick relief to my constant thirst. I'm not saying I now love water or drink as much as I should but I've forced myself to drink more of it and it's not that bad after all, especially when you consider the benefits from something so simple.

Since I'm not a medical professional or have any type of personal experience on this subject, I'll just briefly make this statement and move on. If you have an eating disorder or suspect a loved one has any type of eating disorder, like any health condition, deal with it immediately. It's nothing to be embarrassed or ashamed of. Because I used to vomit for years while at work or even while visiting friends and no one suspected, I know it can be hidden for a long time. However the fact is, because you can hide it doesn't mean you don't need help. Honestly look at your situation, accept the fact something is wrong and get medical help because putting any health condition off, doesn't bring about healing!

Diet adjustments are a lifelong struggle and trust me, adjusting to learn to eat proper portions of all foods is a struggle, at least for me. Develop the mind frame and attitude you're going to adjust your diet and choose realistic expectations so you don't get frustrated and quit because you feel like you've failed. Be aware of what you're eating instead of just grabbing something out of habit and have some type of positive support like a spouse, doctor or mirror. In turn, you'll be able to adjust your diet with more success. The great reward you'll obtain is better overall health and better self-esteem: both of which will improve your overall quality of life and hopefully make continuing your positive life change a reality for years to come.

In regard to self-esteem, don't judge yourself by how others look, but instead on your feelings toward yourself. Don't allow society to program you about how you should look to be beautiful but instead base your appearance goals on how you feel and how you want to look. Realistic goals are the ones you're going to achieve and sometimes life, and your health, will dictate those goals for you.

I grew up thin with well-defined calf muscles as a result of playing so much basketball. I had tons of self-esteem and confidence, almost to the point of being cocky, which showed in the way I carried myself. I loved the way I looked and felt about myself. Then into my life came sarcoidosis, prednisone and other uncontrollable changes! Obviously the way I felt healthwise changed, along with getting older, but my appearance permanently changed as well. Primarily as a result of the prednisone, my weight blew up. My face now has the "round face" look and even today I still at times have to look twice when I pass a mirror. In addition I have a "round stomach", which is shaped in that manner again as a result of prednisone and other medications/factors. If you look closely I resemble a pregnant man. Of course I must take some responsibility as my diet had an impact on the size of my middle whether I blame those other facts of my life or not.

To add to my new look, as a primary result of all of the depo-testosterone injections, my back and shoulders are extremely hairy. I've always had hair on my arms and chest but now I look like one of those men a kid will see at the beach and run like a scared Halloween trick. There's nothing I can do about it since I must get the injections. I'll admit at first I was self-conscious at times when in public, but this is now who I am. On the flip side I've lost my hair on the top of my head, which doesn't run in our family; consequently I keep my hair cut real low to blend together. My legs are bald as well, again as a result of side effects from my medications and aren't well defined as they once were, even when I walk on a regular basis. My looks do at times affect my self-esteem and the fact I don't play basketball anymore still affects my approach to life from a feeling cool or cocky standpoint. I understand why and honestly accept my fate; it's the dealing with it that's tough, as I'm only human.

However I get over it real quick because "I am who I am". I still love myself and my wife loves me as I am as well. "Who cares what anybody else thinks", I tell myself! Changes in your appearance will oc-cur throughout life as a result of aging, health changes and your diet, so you must adjust accordingly. Be your own person! It's normal to have temporary downfalls but remember there are enough things in life trying to bring you down already so don't allow something as artificial as your outside appearance to be another negative force!

Around every corner something awaits to challenge your mental outlook. Major causes of depression certainly would include a chronic health condition with which you or a loved one has been diagnosed as well as other sources such as physical limitations – personal changes – deaths – financial problems – sexual issues – or diet changes. Having a positive outlook and attitude will allow you to be able to deal with a multitude of life situations successfully but depression is always around the next corner to bring you down and is something of which you must be aware in order to adjust. Everyone is different in how they handle depression and depression itself is caused by different sources.

I understand there can be a chemical imbalance in the brain that causes a person to experience severe depression and medications are available to treat the imbalance properly. In fact, I know some people these medications do wonders for when taken correctly. But these types of medications aren't always the answer for everyone. I think too many times medical professionals will not take the time and effort, for whatever reasons, to see what's causing depression in a patient, especially children.

There are many causes for a person to be depressed. Depression could be a result of a side effect of a medication or something in a person's personal life. Sometimes depression is a result of another health condition unrelated to a chemical imbalance. Look at my case. During my many doctors visits in my symptoms stage when I was experiencing migraine headaches on a regular basis, the doctors solution was to try and send me to a psychiatrist because my migraines were in my head (no pun intended). The reality was the migraines were caused by the problem with my vertebrae and sarcoidosis. Same holds true for my sexual issues and other health problems I was experiencing and the doctors weren't taking the time to figure out nor having any success; therefore my symptoms were in my mind. I'm not the only patient I know of where it was suggested they suffered from depression and needed to see a psychiatrist when in reality it was another health issue causing their problems. A lot of times it was sarcoidosis. I beg the medical community to take mental health issues seriously but at the same time don't be so quick to judge. It might be something else. At least take the time to look and if you don't know just honestly say so.

Being a successful patient will not be easy and will run you through a variety of emotions from fear of the unknown to frustration to impatience to guilt to depression to relief. The mental battles will try to wear you down. Don't let them! Use all of the resources you have available to combat those negative forces. Don't let them get the best of you! Use your caregivers, loved ones, support groups, your medical professionals, friends, faith, and most of all your inner voice to help you when you feel you can't make it on your own. We're only human and as humans we can only physically and mentally take so much. Listen to your body and feelings. Learn what your limits are. Accept what your body and mind tells you because there's no one who can tell you better regarding how you feel than your own body and mind. Trust in yourself because you know yourself better than anyone else.

I want to leave you with this thought. Regardless of a person's disability or how many chronic health conditions alter the normalcy of a person's life, the one thing we all want is to be treated with respect, the same as any other person. Granted we might need special assistance to achieve that normalcy, at home or in the workplace, but it's the normalcy that's important to us. Don't give us looks of pity or talk about us as if we aren't there. I once heard some college athletes who happen to participate in wheelchair basketball say the worst thing people would say about them was how much of an inspiration they were for playing basketball in a wheelchair as opposed to giving them the normal credit of being a good athlete. Instead, they only concentrated on their being an inspiration. If you don't understand that logic, stop and take a moment to think seriously about it. As individuals treat us as you would anyone else you encounter, or better yet, treat us how you would want to be treated yourself if the shoes were on the other feet. It's okay for you to be inspired by someone who battles the odds but first give credit for the accomplishments not the inspiration. Normalcy!

Just because a people are disabled or live with chronic health conditions don't mean their emotional needs as human beings, talents and ability to be productive individuals doesn't exist anymore. In fact because of the health conditions those talents might be sharper as more attention is paid to the skill and their desire to achieve has increased. Everyone in this world has something positive to offer. Don't allow your hang-ups or prejudices keep someone else from contributing what they have to offer, especially because they only have a disability, live with chronic health conditions or aren't exactly like you. You'll never know about a person unless you give them an opportunity. You owe providing an open-minded opportunity to yourself because the one person who might make your world complete just might be "that" person with the disability. My wife didn't shy away from me in 1989 because I had health issues and I thank God she didn't!

Let's start concentrating in a positive manner on our similarities and not negatively on our differences. If we must look at our differences, look at them from the standpoint your strength might be my weakness and thus together we can be successful in whatever we put our talents toward. Everyone has something to offer and we need each other to be successful. Patients need their medical professionals to survive and medical professionals need their patients to have a successful practice. Patients need our caregivers while our loved ones need us. Elected officials need their voters to stay in office and voters need their elected officials to be their voice along with their actions to get issues important to us passed into law. Corporations need their customers and employees to have a successful business and consumers need products they can afford and use while employees need jobs to support their families and benefits to ensure they maintain a positive quality of life. Our children need responsible parents to teach and raise them properly into adulthood and our parents need their adult children when they're in their time of need. What goes around – comes around. That's what life is all about!

...15...

There's no place for embarrassment in regard to your health. You have the responsibility to ensure you get the medical help you need by honestly communicating any health issues to your medical professionals. Some things in life are out of our control but most things that impact our fate we do have some control to improve. Always take responsibility for you!

16

No One Is Immune From Cancer

Sometimes life can be just that – life! There are certain things in life that regardless of how prepared you are or how strong you might think you are, those experiences can still be devastating to you. From a health perspective, it doesn't matter if you obtain the vast experience of a "Professional Patient", if you have followed every tip I've provided by way of this book, or if you have done your own extensive research. It doesn't matter if you have prepared yourself for the possibilities or if you are caught completely off guard; the initial results and emotions are basically the same. Life is also about adjusting to those experiences that change aspects of our life immediately and permanently. You must learn how to positively adjust your lifestyle and mindset so that you can maintain a positive quality of life in regard to those aspects of life over which you have no control. Cancer is one of life's experiences that would easily fit into this category! From a personal perspective, my life was about to change forever.

The year 2007 started out good for me from a health perspective. I was walking a regular routine, averaging four times around Northland (a local mall) five days a week. My sugar levels were in range, except for those times I gave in to the craving for a donut or two, and my overall health was consistent. I had a successful routine checkup with my endocrinologist on February 15, 2007. My blood tests came back in range, or close to – nothing out of the norm for my health history. Life was good, but then you know how the reality of life can be.

In June I started experiencing a sharp pain in my left heel whenever I walked. As the month progressed so did the pain. On July 9, 2007, I went to a podiatrist to see what was going on. He found I had a problem with the ligament in my heel. The first option was to have a series of cortisone shots directly into the ligament. However, taking into consideration I was a diabetic and steroids cause sugar levels to rise, he chose option two which consisted of sleeping with a Strassburg sock. The Strassburg sock was basically a night splint. It was a knee high sock with a strap that was connected at the toe and attached at the top of the sock via a loop and Velcro so you could adjust how far you wanted to lift your toes while you sleep. The objective of this process was to stretch the ligament back to normal. The only problem I had with this process was after wearing the sock I would begin to cramp in my calf causing me to have to take the sock off in a matter of a few hours. As a result I just lived with the pain. In fact, I can remember being in New York the end of July and walking the city streets in pain.

Other issues I noticed were spots developing on my right calf and every time I tried to talk I would start to cough. Both of these situations reminded me of my pre-sarcoidosis days and I started getting a little concerned. As the days of July continued to pass I started feeling tired and out of breath after the smallest of activity. My heart would be racing to the point I could literally feel it beating at a fast pace without putting my hand against it. Another concern was my feet, ankles, calves, and just above my knees were starting to retain fluid, swelling, and getting hard. The swelling would be greater at night but you could still see light swelling in the morning as well. I noticed my left hand was also swelling, as my wedding ring was getting tighter, but not my right hand. Finally, after years of putting it off, I had scheduled a colonoscopy for October 2, 2007. I also had another routine checkup scheduled with my endocrinologist on August 23, 2007. By the time my appointment came about I was starting to feel tired most of the time and talking with the constant cough was now a chore. Once again my health was getting weird, or as the doctors say – unusual.

On the day of the appointment, for the first time, my wife decided she should go to the appointment with me, showing she was concerned as well. We told my endocrinologist, who had a couple of interns sitting in on the appointment, everything that was going on. He took my blood pressure and listened to my heart rate and decided to decrease my blood pressure medicine from 20MGs to 10MGs. He also wanted me to get a biopsy on the spots on my calf as my wife brought up the point her mother had similar spots on her legs when she developed cancer. Then most definitely he wanted me to keep this colonoscopy appointment. As always he also did a multitude of blood tests.

A couple of days later I returned home and had a voice mail from my endocrinologist. He had a very serious and stern tone as he told me my blood work showed I was anemic as my white blood cells and hemoglobin levels were low. I remember making a blank statement to my wife whereas I said, "I think sarcoidosis can cause low white blood cells, but so can another disease (referring to cancer although I didn't actually say the "C" word)." She just looked at me without saying a word, but you could see the agreement in her eyes. My endocrinologist suspected I was losing blood somewhere and there were potential problems with my colon and liver. He told me not to go on any out of town trips until we figured out what was going on, as there was a danger I could pass out at anytime, because I had now become anemic. I was to call him the next morning. He knew I had a personal trip with my wife scheduled to New York to celebrate her birthday on September 8, 2007, and I was also scheduled to attend a walk-a-thon, speak, and attend a dinner for a sarcoidosis organization in Houston the end of October. I contacted the leader of the Houston organization and we decided to wait until after the colonoscopy to make an announcement in case I had to cancel, but as far as my personal trip to New York, I was going to do everything in my power to make that trip. However, I would follow my endocrinologist's instructions because my health isn't worth risking for any trip.

I went to see my endocrinologist to plead my case for my New York trip. I told him I knew my body and would seek help or slow down if I felt trouble coming on. I also had spoken at a medical center in the city that at the time had the most cases of sarcoidosis in the country. Plus this was a personal trip, for which I had already paid, and in reality there would be less stress on me there, aside from the actual plane ride. Airport travel in the 21st century is anything but stress free. I told him, with all that said, I would still follow his instructions. The trip was important to me, but my life was more important than any vacation. He listened carefully and reluctantly gave me permission to go.

On the same day as the appointment (September 5, 2007) I got word that a very close friend of mine for whom I had always considered a blood brother passed away, at the age of 49, as a result of a long battle with cancer. This really shook me up because he was starting to do so well. Then, it's my understanding, he woke up one morning and didn't even know who he was. For days he went in and out of a coma until his passing. This was not only a tremendously emotional period for me but once again gave me a personal touch of reality. Rest In Peace, my brother!

The next day, after my endocrinologist appointment, I went to the dermatologist to have a biopsy performed on the spots covering my right calf. It was a simple in-house procedure where the area was deadened then parts of the tissue were removed to be examined in the lab. I should have the results upon my return from New York.

Our New York trip was great! Detroit is my home, and I love it – Perry is my hometown, and I love it – but there is absolutely nowhere on this earth like New York City, and I love it as well! Now in reality, as I've said many times over, it doesn't matter where you go or what new responsibilities you take on, your health is always present – this trip was no different. It was difficult to walk as my feet, ankles, and calves were swollen with water retention. In fact, for the past month or so, I had only one pair of shoes that I could actually wear. I was getting extremely hot (although the weather was absolutely beautiful, but warm), especially when waiting for the subway. In addition my heart was pounding constantly to the point I would get lightheaded. Once again I could literally feel my heart pumping in my chest. In fact, on the night of my wife's birthday (September 8, 2007) I swear I woke up and my heart had stopped for about three seconds, then started racing once again. I lay in bed for a second then got up and sat in a chair until I found a comfortable position. I sat there for about 45 minutes, without moving, while my wife kept asking me if she should call 911 and what medical center should she take me to, although I already had that information written down. Finally I got up and went back to bed, but that experience, I must admit, really scared me for a second.

I took it easy the rest of the trip. We returned to Detroit on September 10, 2007. As I was driving home from the airport I received a call from the dermatologist stating they had received the results from my biopsy. The spots came back as sarcoidosis. To be honest, I was relieved that it was sarcoidosis and not something else. I had her fax the results to my endocrinologist.

The rest of the month I struggled. I was still emotionally upset over the death of my friend and mentally drained from the changes occurring to my body. I was getting more swollen by the day as now my feet, ankles, and legs were swollen up to my thighs. In addition, my left hand had swollen to the point I had to take off my wedding ring, but my right hand remained normal. One thing I hate is to not having my wedding ring on. It's a combination of the little things like this that can have an impact on your overall mental outlook. To top it off the one pair of shoes I had been wearing for the past couple of months were now starting to get harder to put on. I actually had to wear my house shoes at times when I went out in public. I even tried a pair of prescription socks that are supposed to help with circulation; however, they just made things worse as they were extremely tight. I even tried cutting the top of the sock, but that didn't work either. Plus the coughing every time I tried to talk was getting worse and worse. At times I could just take a deep breath and the coughing would start. This was nothing like my pre-sarcoidosis days. No, deep in my heart I knew I was having some major troubles.

I had an appointment and injection due on September 27, 2007, with my endocrinologist so I figured I could wait to talk to him. The morning of the appointment was rough. I had tried to do a couple of minor tasks around the house but as usual was out of breath quickly. I lay down on the bed and not only was I hot and lightheaded, but my heart was beating at a very fast rate, to the point I could literally feel every beat pounding inside my chest. As I lay in bed I seriously thought about calling 911 but the phone was on the television and my cellular phone was on my dresser so I figured I could wait it out as I had been doing for months. Fortunately, and stupidly on my part, I drove myself to my appointment.

When I arrived at the office, the nurse took one look at me and immediately called me from the waiting room. The nurse went ahead and gave me my depo- testosterone injection then my endocrinologist came in. He looked at me and asked in concern, "What is going on with you today?" I told him how I felt and his immediate response was, "You are going to the ER. Do you want me to call an EMS unit or your wife? I've been trying to figure out how I could get you admitted to the hospital with your insurance (never forget it is your insurance that drives most medical decisions these days and it is still wrong), but now I have more than enough reasons." I told him to call my wife to come get me. In the meantime he called my PCP, which, even though

I never see him, is the doctor who must admit me.

My wife soon arrived and we headed to the Emergency Room. When I arrived I was taken back rather quickly because the status of my health condition had been called in. As always the nurse had some connection with my endocrinologist. It seems everyone has been treated by him at one time and there is always the highest praise for him. This, along with my relationship with him, is a major reason I have complete trust in his advice and actions.

I was taken back to a bed where, after answering the same questions a few times to interns and the ER doctor, a team of cardiologists invaded my curtain drawn room. Turns out I was having Congestive Heart Failure with a heart rate of 197. Keep in mind the normal heart rate should be under 100 and anything over 120 is considered a danger zone – mine was steady at 197; I was in a serious situation to say the least. They tried several medications but nothing seemed to slow it down. In addition, when your heart rate races like this your blood pressure drops to danger levels as well. Finally they gave me a medication that would slow my heart to basically not beating for about 5 seconds so the doctors could get a look at what was really going on. The ER doctor told me it would feel like I was driving 100 miles per hour then all of a sudden come to a complete stop. He even counted down the seconds as to when it was going to stop. What a weird and scary feeling those 5 seconds were! They determined my irregular heart beat had gone into what's called atrial fibrillation or fluttering of the heart. One of the doctors's told me it was amazing to her how I could even walk, much less survive for the past month. Eventually, they were able to get the heart rate down to around 140 before they admitted me into the hospital. This turned out to be a long stay!

While in the hospital my heart rate went back to normal on its own, or at least normal for me. Tests showed that my heart was okay, except for the right side being enlarged due to sleep apnea and irregular heartbeat. However, other issues came to light. My endocrinologist was sending all of the top specialists, or Chief-Of- Staffs, to see me, including a pulmonologist and his team. They determine I had a collapsed right lung with fluid surrounding the lung. I went through a procedure where I sat on the side of the bed leaning over the bed tray next to my bed while the doctor put a tube in my back leading to the right lung.

He then proceeded to withdraw two liters of fluid from the outside of my lung. Actually the procedure sounds worse than it was. Except for the poke to deaden the area the only thing I felt was pressure and then I could breathe better. After a few days the coughing went away and I was able to ramble on once again, as my wife says I do.

In regard to my swollen feet, ankles, calves, thighs, and left hand, I was given a medication (Lasik) to eliminate the fluid, along with reducing my intake of DDAVP, the drug to treat my diabetes insipidus. This was a tricky solution because the medications contradicted each other. The Lasik would cause water to leave my body while as the DDAVP's purpose was to retain water. Eventually the Lasik won out.

I also had an ultrasound performed on my legs. As a result of the ultrasound a couple of blood clots were found in my calves. To prevent the blood clots from getting into my lungs, which could cause stroke or death, a Green Filter was implanted in the main artery in my chest leading to my lungs. A Green Filter is basically a metal like umbrella type filter that if a blood clot tried to get to my lungs the Green Filter would dissolve the blood clot, thus preventing it from reaching the lungs. It was an easy procedure where they go through your groin and push the filter into place. I don't even know it's there.

On October 2, 2007, came the big test – a colonoscopy. Except for the preparation the previous night, and you just can't sugarcoat that experience, colonoscopies aren't really that bad. You are in a sleep mode, although I did wake up for a second while the procedure was still going on, and before you know it the doctor is talking to you. For me, this was the part I had feared. With my wife by my side, he looked us straight in the eyes and said, "We found a golf ball size tumor in your colon that is cancer. We also suspect it has spread to your liver but a biopsy must be performed to conclude that determination. I have also sent off a sample of the colon tumor to the lab. An oncologist will see you soon. I'm sorry for the bad news. If there is anything I can do, just let me know." I was then taken back to my room.

Once back in my hospital bed I started to cry as my wife held me and cried with me. The news was not a surprise because, as I said earlier, low white blood cell counts are a possible sign of cancer. Plus there were the same spots on my calves that my mother-in-law developed when she had cancer. Although they came back as sarcoidosis, they had planted the seed in my mind of the possibility of cancer. The diagnosis wasn't a real surprise – but still, there is nothing that can describe the feeling you have when a doctor tells you that you have cancer!

Over the years I've been told by doctors that I would die if nothing was done, that if things continue as they were I would never reach 50, and that I should live everyday as if it were my last because with my health conditions, it could easily be. The fact is, and I'm not trying to be macho, with my unconditional faith I've never been, nor am I now, afraid of death. I'm afraid of pain, but not death, because I know I'm going to a paradise of peace. On the other hand, as a human being, I'm not quite ready to die. I still have things I want to do and I surely am not ready to leave my wife. But now I had Stage 4 cancer and the possibility of my death was real, after all, death is Stage 5!

Cancer is a powerful word! It can bring a multitude of emotions to which everyone can relate, either by way of having cancer themselves or someone close to them has dealt with the disease. When I was diagnosed with sarcoidosis, and even today, I usually have to first explain what sarcoidosis is, and then how it causes the multitude of chronic health conditions. Most times people usually walk away still not understanding. However, when I mention I have cancer, regardless with whom I am talking, they will immediately tell me their story. Everyone has a cancer story, either it is about themselves or someone they know.

In life very seldom do your decisions only affect just you. This is a perfect example. I was originally scheduled to have a colonoscopy performed back in early 2004. You are supposed to stop taking baby aspirin seven days before the procedure so your blood will clot more effectively. When it came time for the colonoscopy I had forgotten – an honest mistake – to stop taking my baby aspirin; therefore the doctor would not do the procedure and I had to reschedule. When it was time for my second appointment my father had just been diagnosed with cancer so I cancelled the colonoscopy and went to Florida. For the next three years I simply made one excuse after another to avoid the procedure. So in reality the fact I wasn't diagnosed with colon cancer until it had reached the last stage is no one's fault but my own. The thing is my decision has touched others because when my life changes or ends, my family's lives will also change forever.

For the next couple of days my wife and I cried together and alone. I started thinking about everything you could possibly think of. I thought about the after life, because no one really knows what happens to your soul. Do I go to a place where I will see my father again, along with everyone else I knew? Will I now know the truth to everything that happened in life while on earth? Will I be able to watch over my mother, wife, daughter, and granddaughter as a guardian angel with powers to improve their lives on earth? Or will I just be in a peaceful deep sleep waiting to come back as something else and find the answer to that one question we have all asked ourselves at some point when doing something we have never done or being someplace we have never been, "Why is this so familiar?", or will I just have a new life? When you're told you have cancer, in the beginning, you feel you are close to finding out.

I also looked back on my life and I'm proud to say I have no regrets. Sure there are some things I would have done differently or wish had turned out better, but the fact is that's only because I now know the outcome. Anyone can make better decisions in hindsight. For me, if I had it to do all over again, I would do it all the same. Finally the day of acceptance came.

It was the morning of October 4, 2007. My wife had just left the hospital around 8:00 AM, after spending the night with me. When she left I again just broke down, and I'm not an emotional guy but crying is a natural reaction to being told you, or a loved one, has cancer. About the time I stopped crying my daughter called to check on me. When I hung up the phone I again broke down. One of the nurses came in and told me I had nothing scheduled this morning and she would close the curtain around my bed. She said she would keep everyone away from me and to call her if I needed anything. For two and a half hours I prayed and meditated; I was angry, depressed, thankful, and hopeful. I thought about every aspect of my life, past and present and I prayed for a future. Cancer might beat me in the end, but cancer was not going to destroy the life I still had in me!

By the time it was all said and done, I had a peaceful feeling inside that was so surreal and I had come to the realization that I had no control over what was going to happen in the end. God was in complete control and my faith still remained unconditional. Don't get me wrong, I still have my moments, as does my wife, but from that time on I was at peace with whatever the future held.

On October 6, 2007, I was finally released from the hospital with a biopsy scheduled on October 10th, as an outpatient to confirm that cancer was in my liver. On October 15th, I got a call from my endocrinologist to confirm that the results from the biopsy showed I had cancer in my liver, as well as my colon. He had already setup an appointment with the oncologist for October 17th, to go over the game plan, which consists of chemotherapy sessions starting October 24th.

At this time I also had an epiphany that only grandparents can experience that gave me the inspiration to live at least long enough for my 19-month-old granddaughter to be able to remember me. Let me tell you a little story as to why being a grandfather is so special. When I was in the hospital I told my daughter not to bring my grandbaby to the hospital, but since she wanted to check on me and had no one to keep the baby, she brought her to the room a couple of times. Each time she was okay, although she never came up to the bed, and when she got ready to leave she would wave goodbye. But when my daughter would ask her to give PaPa a kiss she would start crying. The day I was released they also came by the house. As I was in bed the same situation occurred where she was okay but would burst out crying when my daughter tried to have her kiss me goodbye.

A few days later I was in bed and heard my daughter and granddaughter in the next room. By now the swelling had gone down in my legs and hand (most of it that is) and I was starting to get my strength back. I walked into the room and as soon as my granddaughter looked at me, she stopped eating, and ran up to me and said, "PaPa." I told her that one of her doll's shoes, for which we had been looking, was in the living room and we walked to get the shoe. Once she got the shoe she threw it down and lifted her arms for me to pick her up, saying, "PaPa, PaPa!" I picked her up and usually she will look around but this time she immediately put her arms around my neck real tight and buried her head in my shoulder, as if thinking PaPa is back. It was the warmest feeling I have ever known. After a few minutes, and the fact I was getting tired (she is getting heavier) I wiped the tears from my eyes and tried to put her down. As she reached the floor she tightened her grip around my next and still never lifted her head from my shoulder.

I held her another minute or so then took her back to the room where my wife and daughter were sitting. When we entered the room my granddaughter let go and went back to her normal busy self. At that moment she became my primary inspiration to live!

Before the chemotherapy session I was scheduled to have a single Picc Line inserted into my left arm on October 19, 2007. A Picc Line is basically an IV that is run into the main artery in your arm and is used for chemotherapy, IV medications, and drawing blood. However, that night I started running a fever and ended up spending three nights in the hospital once again.

My chemotherapy session consisted of several medications given to me via my Picc Line and lasted about four hours. Then I was given a fusion box that provides constant chemotherapy for 48 hours. I also received an injection the following day after the fusion box was removed to increase my white blood cells. The first chemotherapy session didn't go as planned.

I felt good until the end of the session when I started to have diarrhea. The problem was the diarrhea wasn't stools but blood. The oncologist told me when I got home if I continued to have blood diarrhea to go to the ER immediately. I got home and after about an hour I had another case of blood diarrhea. Stubborn Gil went back to bed instead of the ER. In about 30 minutes it hit me again, only harder. As I was sitting on the toilet having blood continue to flow from my rectum, I could not move as I went in and out of even knowing where I was. My wife called EMS and the next thing I knew I was in the hospital for another three days. My oncologist determined it was one of the medications that was supposed to shoot massive quantities of blood to the colon to reduce the tumor. Instead it just messed me up! Once we stopped that particular medication I didn't have that specific problem again.

Chemotherapy can be rough from both a physical and mental aspect on any individual and his/her loved ones. Although we are all unique and side effects affect each of us differently, including how our loved ones accept the side effects, there are many situations that we all experience. Chronic fatigue is probably the worst, both from a physical and mental perspective. When talking with other chemotherapy patients I found that the inability to follow their normal routine because of tiredness affected their mental outlook more than the physical issues. One advantage I have in this scenario is the fact I have been dealing with chronic fatigue for over 20 years. Although with the chemotherapy I have insomnia and sleep during the morning whereas with the chronic fatigue relating to my sarcoidosis I can sleep anytime (I've even fallen asleep standing up). I try to give positive advice to the other patients on how I learned to accept my reality in regard to the emotions of laziness, uselessness, helplessness, and the feelings of letting others down, including myself, as a result of chronic fatigue. The only problem with my advice is it took me a few years before I honestly came to grips with dealing with chronic fatigue whereas these patients don't have years to understand – they need to deal with it in a positive manner right now.

Other side effects that years ago were more common are nausea, diarrhea, and constipation. Don't get me wrong, these side effects are still present, and at times can not only be a life changing experience, but painful as well. It's just that in today's environment there are preventive medications used to prevent these side effects and if they do occur there are better medications to treat them causing them to be less severe, although still uncomfortable. The old days of patients bent over the toilet for hours after a chemotherapy session are "pretty much" a thing of the past, but again we are all different.

Then there are the other varieties of side effects such as loss of hair, loss of appetite and loss of sexual drives as well as sensitivity to the sun, mood swings, depression and the list goes on. Like with any chronic health conditions you must do what you can as a patient, with hopefully the help of a loved one, to understand what you "might" expect in regard to side effects, understanding that you "might" not experience them all, if any. Don't forget the 3-Step Philosophy!

Personally, my side effects have included insomnia (especially on the night I receive the chemotherapy) along with chronic fatigue, thinning of my body hair, sore bones as a result of medication, and a routine of three days of constipation or diarrhea along with a white chalk like coating of my tongue starting Thursday (while on the chemotherapy fusion box) until the following Tuesday when it is completely gone. During this time there is an awful taste in my mouth as well. Then in a week it's time to start the process all over again. I have noticed as the number of sessions increase, the side effects get more intense and the mental battle becomes tougher. But what choice do you have but to deal with it in the best manner you can?

When it comes to dealing with life my wife and I are a perfect team, even if we do get on each other's nerves from time to time. Some might think we are weird or off the wall in our philosophies on how we handle things but I think those people just try to make things too complicated. Life, including dealing with chronic health conditions, is really a series of simple processes, as we have already discussed in the book. Not easy – just simple.

When I came to grips with my situation I made the decision that I was going to eliminate all possible negativity and drama from my life, with the help of my wife. I did not want to be in communication with anyone who was going to be depressed about my situation or bring drama to the table…period! Let me explain this so you will understand my point of view. First of all, I understand the first time I break the news to someone it is going to be emotional. I understand this and except this fact, that's not what I'm talking about. I cried with many of my friends and family the first time the news was broke.

I'm talking about dealing with those individuals who after several conversations still are crying or feeling sorry for you. They look at you with sad eyes and pity. Don't need it!!! Then there are those who are just drama queens and drama kings. Again, don't need it!!! Only positive energy is going to be around me during this time. If it hurts someone's feelings, so be it. Ask me this – would I rather hurt someone who brings negativity and drama into my life causing stress which consequently brings on additional health problems or would I rather not let those into my life who would cause harm because of their situation or just their personalities? The answer is obvious, at least to my wife and me. Remember when dealing with cancer and chemotherapy you are in a life and death situation where your survival and quality of life is in your hands. You must under any circumstance, whether it offends or not, stay positive and do what is best for you. In other situations, yes, you may look the other way and, except for being irritated, little harm is done. However, in this case, a little harm can cause time off my life. There comes a point in life when you must become the number one priority, and accept that fact. Otherwise? How about we skip the otherwise!

You also have to remember and recognize that people deal with other people's health conditions, along with death, in different ways. Cancer is a prime example. I have a perfect support structure in place that works for me. First, is my wife who I know without a doubt has my back in all situations. She will get me what I need, ensure I get the proper medical treatment, give me freedom to do what I can while at the same time does not hesitate to get on me when I'm doing too much, even if it makes me mad, and keeps the negativity/drama away from me. The part that hurts me is she must also take up some of my former responsibilities I have trouble doing based on my health situation. Although I think it showed her how spoiled I had made her, it really hurts me inside to have to watch her do the simple things I should be doing in our relationship. Hey, no one said facing, then accepting reality was easy, no matter how many times you've had to do it. My wife has a good support structure by way of her employer and friends who are willing to help out if needed, even if it's just to lend a listening ear.

Secondly, I have my daughter who constantly checks on me to see if she can do anything. I tell her the best thing she can do is to take care of her own business, school, and my grandbaby so that her mother and I don't have to worry about her. I tell her not to worry about me but as we all know those are just words as the next day she is calling again. Hey, I understand as I call my mother almost everyday as well. My mother, although she lives in Florida, is another of my support pillars. Even though I worry about her more than myself, she still provides encouraging words and just knowing her unconditional love is waiting on me at anytime is enough to turn a negative day into a positive one. In addition I have a couple of men living in Perry who have been like brothers to me my entire life. One calls on a regular basis. I kid him that he is going to drive me crazy with his overprotective worrying about me, just like my wife and mother. Don't get me wrong, I'm just joking around because I love them all to death. The other also calls and the good part is, from past experiences, I know he would do anything I needed him to do at anytime. Those are true blood brothers! Then there are other friends who call or e-mail checking up on me and providing positive words. Of course, there are those who don't know what to say, even when they do call, so I don't hear from them as often as I might like. It's not surprising because the same has happened in the past and I'm not a phone caller myself, but still sometimes you expect more from those who are supposed to be close to you. But then when you already know what you're dealing with it doesn't bother you enough to cause negative vibes – you just blow it off. People are who they are!

Another great source of support for me are the many, many, many folks around the world who sent me cards, letters, and e-mails when I was first diagnosed. It made me feel good to know I had made such an impact on others' lives. When you are just going about your everyday business most readers, or people for that matter, don't bother sending thank you cards or let you know the positive impact your story had on their lives (the ones that hated your books will, but not usually the positive ones). This meant a lot to me and helped me rise above my negative outlook. However, the most important thing they, and everyone else, gave me was their prayers. The power of prayer is important to me and I believe it does make a difference. So to all of those who have prayed for me I say from the bottom of my heart – you could not have given me a better gift and I thank you!

Last, but not least, my greatest inspiration is my (at the time of this writing) 2 year and 10 month-old granddaughter. As I said earlier, my short-term goal is to live long enough for her to remember me. I don't know what age that is, but I want her to be able to look at a picture of us and describe what was going on, as opposed to looking at the same picture and having someone else tell her the story. Every time I look at her or hold her it brings such a warm feeling to my heart. I have a lot of other reasons to want to live, people whom I love, and things I still want to do, but my granddaughter is my inspiration – no doubt about it.

Everyone in a life and death or quality of life situation needs to have positive motivation in order to continue to deal with their health situation. Never underestimate that power of positive support and your own positive outlook. Sure, there are bad days, I know I have quite a few, but you must always try and find a positive in those bad days because in every situation there is a positive – you just have to find it.

Other good resources are support groups or studies. We participated in a study for cancer patients and their caregivers in which you are given surveys and visits from nurses to see how you are doing and what you need. The study really helped us, but not in the way you may think. We had four in-home visits and one conference call and each time the nurses were amazed at how in touch my wife and I are not only with each other, but also with the battles we are facing. We were on the same page with the answers we provided (separately) and the honesty with which we communicate. We didn't sugarcoat our feelings or situations thus allowing us to deal with them in a positive manner with positive results. Both nurses said we were such a positive and unique couple and there was really no advice or material they could provide us that we weren't already doing. I think the fact I have always had chronic health conditions and my wife had cancer before I did plays a major factor in how we are handling my cancer experience. Don't get me wrong, it is hard and emotional! Real hard and emotional! But with the right attitude, support, and faith – anyone can overcome!

My next three chemotherapy sessions went well. After the fourth we did a CT Scan to determine if the treatment was working. It wasn't exactly the report I was looking for. My oncologist came in and told us that there was no change in the tumor or liver, as he was hoping there would be. He seemed kind of down about the results. Actually, this was a perfect Catch 22 if there ever was one. On the glass-half-empty outlook you can say that nothing changed therefore the chemotherapy isn't doing the job to reduce and kill the cancer for which you had hoped. On the glass-half-full outlook (the approach I took) you can say that nothing changed therefore the tumor hasn't grown so the chemotherapy is doing something. Even though I have obviously taken a step down in regard to my quality of life I can still live a productive fulfilling life if everything stays the same. I was also having major hemorrhoid problems and had recently seen the doctor who performed the colonoscopy. He gave me a few tips on how to keep the hemorrhoids down such as soaking in a warm sitz bath, using a warm rolled up wash cloth to put on the hemorrhoids, preferably with a heating pad as well, and gave me a prescription for a stronger cream to use directly on them. He also wanted to see the results of my CT Scan as he was hoping the tumor would shrink so he could go in and cut it out. My oncologist told me that probably wouldn't happen as he said, "Surgeons are always more optimistic and just look at operating while oncologists are used to dealing with bad news and are more realistic." Therefore, our current plan was to continue as is for four more treatments then we would test again.

The next four treatments went okay, I guess. It started getting harder from a physical standpoint after each session and then when I finally got myself together it was time to start all over again. I was still able to cope and do most of the things I wanted to do but by the time the eighth chemotherapy session was over on February 6, 2008, I was a happy man and ready to see what results we were going to get on February 13, 2008. Plus I had my first trip scheduled since all of this cancer stuff began so I was going to be able to skip my next session which should give my body time to recover from all of these drugs. My wife and I were going to take our 23-month-old granddaughter to Florida to visit my mother for a week and at the same time I would turn 50-years-old myself on February 28, 2008. I had really been looking forward to this trip and nothing was going to stop me from going. But you know how life can throw you a challenge. Here comes another one!

On February 11, 2008 I got my CT Scan early that morning. Everything went well, except I was feeling tired and lightheaded. When I got home I made a few phone calls regarding taking our car in for repair due to us being involved in an accident on February 8, 2008. A truck pulled out in front of us. While we were in the left lane he decided to try and come from the right lane and turn onto an exit for which he had already passed, not to mention the roads were icy, then he stopped in front of us so my wife ran into the side of his truck. As I hung up the phone with my insurance agent I walked upstairs to get ready to take the car to the repair shop and pick up a rental car. When I put on my coat I started to feel real lightheaded and hot. Those tingles you get just before you vomit started to make their presence known. I was also yawning (a sign your body is trying to get oxygen) and I was getting dizzy. I figured I better go sit on the loveseat in our living room and let things get back to normal before I left home. As I approached the loveseat the next thing I knew I was falling to the floor. I got up and threw my coat on the sofa and sat down still experiencing all of the above feelings.

I took out my cellular phone and called my wife at work (she is always the first one I think to call). As soon as she heard my voice she asked what was wrong. I told her that I had just fallen but didn't lose consciousness. She told me to open the front door (a few step from where I was seated) and she was calling 911. I made it to the door and back to the loveseat. I remember I was seeing blurry as my front window was all light and I couldn't see the traffic passing by our house. I wanted to get a towel to wipe the sweat from my head but couldn't make myself get up. I knew something was just not right about this situation!

The next thing I know there were about six EMS people in my living room. The head technician sat on the sofa and started talking to me while a couple of technicians were checking my vitals and another was checking my sugar levels. I told the head technician what happened and I didn't want to go to the ER because they would just admit me again and I hated being in the hospital. He told me, "Mr. Barr I won't kidnap you against your will" in a laughing tone, although I noticed his head was facing me but his eyes were looking, with concern, at the other technicians. The next thing I knew he said, "Mr. Barr I can't leave you home alone" and two of the technicians were moving my loveseat, grabbed me around the legs and chest and took me outside to the waiting stretcher. I told the head technician to lock my house and where to find the keys. As I was being put into the EMS unit I noticed both of my sleeves were rolled up and my shirt was lifted up as well exposing my stomach. Keep in mind it was about six degrees with a wind chill factor of minus 15. I looked at the head technician and asked, "Shouldn't I at the very least be cold right now?" He smiled and replied, "Probably, I know I am." The fact was I was still burning up inside.

I was rushed to the nearby medical center (about five minutes from my home) as they called ahead a Code One. I was immediately taken to the Trauma Unit and a nurse and doctor immediately went to work on me (this had never happened before). After about an hour I was sent to the Chest Pain Unit with a heart rate staying steady between 155 and 190 as my blood pressure continued to drop to dangerous levels. Once again I was experiencing a Congestive Heart Failure with an atrial fibrillation, which if not controlled can cause a high risk of stroke or even death.

As the cardiologists continued to try medication after medication, with no success, the decision was made by the Chief Of Staff to give me electric shock treatment. At this time I realized this was a serious situation! Electric shock treatment is where they place a pad on both your chest and back and shoot shock waves into your heart to cause it to stop for a few seconds. The objective is that your heart will start back at its normal rate. I guess you could say they were jump starting my heart. Of course like with any procedure there is always the chance my heart would not start back correctly or at all, again causing a high risk of stroke or possible death. Fortunately for me, the procedure went as planned and when I was awakened my heart rate was between 95 and 110. I spent the night in the Cardiac Intensive Care Unit and was released the next day. My blood pressure medication was stopped and I was given another medication to control the rhythm of my heart rate. I also plan on getting a procedure that will stop the atrial fibrillation in March or April so hopefully I can, and my wife as well, stop worrying about when my heart will switch into a flutter.

The next day, February 13, 2008, I went to my oncologist to get the results of my CT Scan. Once again the report was the same – no change. He went on to explain that he really couldn't get a good look at the tumor in my colon unless we did a colonoscopy, which he wasn't going to do at this time. Also as far as my liver goes he couldn't tell the difference between the granulomas (sarcoidosis), cysts, or cancer, although we do know cancer is present by way of the biopsy. As long as everything looked the same then that was a good thing. His overall attitude this time around, although the results were the same, was positive. I asked him, "Is this a good thing?" for which he replied, "Yes, it's a good thing!" with a smile on his face. So for now we are going to just keep doing what we are doing and put our faith in God.

One thing I am going to do with all my power is stay out of the hospital as much as I can. Let me give you some insider info on being in the hospital, or at least the medical center I'm always in. First of all, you do not go to the hospital for rest – you go to get well. Someone is always coming in on you to draw blood, get your vitals, give you medications, and everything else under the sun. Do not expect to just lie back and rest. Next, expect to answer the same questions over and over again to nurses, residents, interns, fellows, and doctors. And if you have a unique health condition like I do, expect even more visitors. Just remember you don't have to answer to everyone. If you get tired of being asked the same questions ask to speak to your doctor and let him/her know of your frustrations. They'll call off the inquisitive minds.

Another real frustration and this might not be true for all medical centers, but it sure is true for the one I stay in – the food is terrible! It is barely edible, and I'm not exaggerating as everyone I asked tells me the same thing. They will come and get your order then won't even give you what you asked for. I got coffee everyday even though everyday I told them I didn't drink coffee. Now this is more than an inconvenience, it can do the patient harm. For example, a roommate of mine, who was a diabetic, received a meal with coffee and five packs of sugar along with ice cream, not something a diabetic who is in the hospital as a result of his sugar levels should be given to eat. I remember being in this same medical center in 1991 and 2005 and at that time the food was good. They've changed vendors and now, well, it's just nasty. Not all medical centers are this bad from a food perspective, or so I've been told. Just keep in mind you're not going to get a home cooked meal, at least at most medical centers.

Here is one of the things that gets to me the most regarding being in the hospital. The pharmacy/staff gives you your medications based on their schedule as opposed to when you normally are scheduled to take your medications. I understand this is better for them to have a standard schedule but there is a reason why patients take their medications at a certain time. I could give you too many examples so I'll just give you one that shows my point. I take my insulin at meals based on my current blood sugar reading. In other words if my sugar is over 150 I take 18 units of insulin – if my sugar is over 200 I take 20 units – and so on. Each morning the nurse will take my sugar reading at 6:00 AM but yet breakfast doesn't come till 8:30 AM, at which time, based on their schedule, they don't retake it. By that time my sugar could be 50 points higher or lower, but yet we are basing my meal insulin amount on a reading two and a half hours earlier. I even had one nurse who was going to give me my insulin at 6:00 AM as well. Doesn't make sense to me! In addition, certain medications are given at only certain times, such as my blood thinner is only given at 6:00 AM regardless of when the patient takes it at home. The patient is not a scheduling thing, but a patient and there is a reason why their doctor has them taking medications at a certain time.

One positive thing that I've experienced this time around from my previous visits is the knowledge and attention given to my sarcoidosis. It is like night and day from when I was previously in the ER or medical center. From the specialist to the ER doctor if they weren't sure of something they asked. I only had one ER doctor who when I told her she needed to call my endocrinologist she replied, "My whole family has diabetes and I probably will too one day so I know a lot about diabetes." Needless to say I was uncomfortable with her and looked for someone else very quickly. But overall I saw a positive improvement in the awareness of sarcoidosis and how it affects the body. That was good to see!

Another thing I want to mention regarding hospital stays is if you are a visitor, other than immediate family, please only stay five or ten minutes. The person you are visiting probably loves to see you but they are sick and in the hospital, not for a social visit but to get well. Some folks come and stay for hours while the family is too polite to tell them to leave. When you are in the hospital your health is top priority, not a social visit. Please keep this in mind the next time you visit a friend in the hospital – if you aren't asked to stay longer then never stay longer than 10 minutes. You will be doing everyone a favor!

My last issue is one I know hospitals and insurance companies are going to balk at, but here goes – I feel all rooms that patients are admitted to during hospital stays should be private rooms. Not just for the rich and famous, but for everyone. I know the hospitals feel it will cause them to not be able to admit as many patients, although if the design is done correctly this is not true. They may also complain that it will take more staff, but again if the leaders, who do get paid big bucks for their knowledge and foresight, set it up right then this can be worked out as well. I am aware of one major Detroit medical center (unfortunately not the one I use) whose goal is to have all patient rooms private in the future. Of course the insurance companies will balk because they seem to balk at everything.

Now here are the advantages as to why I feel private rooms should be required. First is the fact that when you are in the hospital, regardless of how clean the staff keeps the facility and themselves, there are germs everywhere, just based on the fact the hospital is filled with sick people. Adding to the problem is having two sick people in the same room, side by side. You have no idea what the patient next to you has or how it might interact/interfere with what you are experiencing and in turn make you sicker. Especially patients on chemotherapy, have sarcoidosis or any other health conditions that weakens the immune system. It simply makes medical sense to not have two patients living together with two different diseases and two different physical/mental make-ups. Then you have the visitors who, once again, you have no idea what kind of conditions or common colds they might have to share. It just doesn't make medical healing sense! Germs should be kept to themselves, not spread around freely!

Secondly is the privacy issue. When doctors or family members are with the patient everything discussed is heard by the other patient in the room, and their visitors. After all, there is only a curtain separating the patients and it's not like you can ask the other patient to step out of the room for a few minutes, so every word, regardless of how low you talk, is heard by someone you don't even know, much less want to know your most private medical details and hear your private emotions. Isn't that the basis of the HIPAA medical privacy policy? A doctor cannot talk about your health condition in a public place and doctor's offices are putting up shields at their check in desk so others cannot see other patients medical paperwork or hear discussions while in the waiting room, but yet your most private medical discussions in your hospital bed between you and your doctor, along with the private emotions that follow, can be heard word for word by complete strangers - your hospital roommate and their visitors. Things, information, and emotions you might want to keep from family members or close friends are openly heard by strangers who we all know go home and tell their family and friends about what they heard – that's just human nature. Tell me…what kind of logic is that?

Last is the comfort element which speeds up the healing process. First is the patient who now, although woke up constantly for his/her own requirements, doesn't have to be woke up for his/her roommate's as well since the light always is turned on and conversations persist. The patient also doesn't have to deal with the little, but annoying, things such as snoring, coughing, sounds of pain, the TV on, unwanted conversation, etc. This allows the patient to get what little rest they can, and more of it, thus helping the healing process.

In addition, comfortable chairs or a sofa should be available for the visitors. It makes me feel so guilty to see my wife sitting so uncomfortable for hours on end while I am in the hospital or getting chemotherapy. The family's comfort should be considered as well and with a private room, along with comfortable seating, the family member can stay longer, overnight if they choose, without being miserable. This will again help the mental state of the patient and thus speed up recovery. News flash – the faster the patient recovers the more patients a hospital can admit and money insurance companies save! In my opinion, this is something that should seriously be considered.

The remaining of 2008 has seen my cancer and other chronic health conditions pretty much stay stable as I continue to get chemotherapy treatments every other week. I was able to take my wife and granddaughter to Florida to visit my mother for my 50th birthday on February 28th – a milestone some thought I would never see – but once again I proved them wrong. That was a very special trip to me and a time I will always cherish. When you are in my current health situation you cherish every moment even more, as in a perfect world you should anyway regardless of your health situation.

I had one issue where I dehydrated based on the fact I got a virus bug and was not drinking the fluids I was supposed to such as Gatorade. Sound familiar? I had to be given fluids via a two hour IV and was told to start drinking my fluids, especially Gatorade, immediately and regularly. You would have thought I would have learned from my father. I guess we all have a little hypocrite in us as it is easier to tell others what to do than do it ourselves. I've learned my lesson! In addition, I have had a couple of other health issues which required hospital stays during 2008.

The first was in March 2008 when my feet, ankles, then legs, started to swell along with turning a purple color. Walking became something I couldn't do more than a few yards without having to stop and rest. The reason for the swelling turned out to be several blood clots had clogged my Green Filter in my main artery thus forcing the blood flow to my legs to find another route, which wasn't very successful. Hey, at least the Green Filter did its job and stopped the blood clots from reaching my lungs and causing my death!

I was started on daily 150MG injections of a blood thinner which unclogged the Green Filter allowing the blood to once again flow to my legs and the swelling reduced. I think I still get blood clots from time to time but overall, except for my feet and legs slightly swelling and cramping, the blood thinner is doing the job. I spent a night in the hospital just for precautionary measures.

The other came in November 2008 when my atrial fibrillation kicked in again as my heart rate was steady around 160. I had not had the procedure to treat this condition done as planned due to the doctor wanted me to be in this state when the procedure was performed.

This was not a very good hospital experience as I went to the emergency room around 3:00 PM on Sunday afternoon and on Monday morning around 8:00 AM I still had not spoken to the doctor nor were my other doctors called, even though I kept telling everyone who needed to be called. Finally my wife and I spoke to my primary physician and told him our frustration level had been reached. He left to make some phone calls and returned to tell me the specialist was at another hospital but would stop by to see me before midnight – this was at around 8:30 AM! They were giving me medication which would lower the heart rate for about 15 minutes then it would return to the 160 range. We told him this was unacceptable because I was previously told if I went into fibrillation again he would have me on the operating table within a couple of hours, plus the last time I had fibrillation and the medication did the same thing they were giving me electric shock treatments within four hours and now no one seems to be concerned. See me before midnight?!

In a few minutes my endocrinologist (who should always be called and I had not only told them several times but it is on my medical sheet I always provide) happened to be on the floor and came in. He immediately ordered my stress steroids which are needed due to my sarcoidosis effect and once again I had been telling the nurses and doctors all night. I was allowed to eat lunch around 11:00 AM but around 1:00 PM they came in to take me to have my procedure performed (you aren't supposed to eat after midnight the night before when you are going to be put under due to the acid in your stomach having possible bad interaction with the medications used to put you under during the procedure). I have to assume someone finally actually talked to the specialist who knew the urgency of the matter. Around 3:30 PM I was on the operating table and the procedure, where they entered my neck and burnt off the part of the heart that was causing problems, was performed. By 9:00 PM that same evening I was at home eating dinner and sleeping in my own bed. It was the best night's sleep I had in months!

As I have stressed many times you must stand up for your rights as a patient and it makes it even better to have someone with you who can, and will, stand up for you when you can't. If we had never spoken up then who knows what might have happened. I don't understand why the quality of service from the emergency room staff to the nurses to the pharmacy (once again I didn't get the medications I should have and the ones I did were not at the time I should have) to the doctors (other than my own) was the way it was this visit. In fact, the next time I saw my oncologist, a couple of days later, he didn't even know I had been in the hospital or had the procedure, although I was told by the emergency room doctor and nurse he was going to be called. I did complain to the follow-up call I received from the hospital but I got the feeling the caller didn't want to hear what I had to say and actually asked me if I wanted him to tell anyone at the hospital. Duh!!! I just don't understand what was the problem this trip? Fortunately everything has worked out and my heart rate and blood pressure has remained under control.

I received my last CT Scan on December 8, 2008 and once again my condition remains the same. The tumor is still the same size in the colon and some of the spots (sarcoidosis or cancer) have slightly decreased. The positive result is no new growths or spots have been detected. Although I cannot sugarcoat the harsh reality of being on chemotherapy for 14 months, with no end in sight, life goes on and that's what's really important. My oncologist can't explain why I am reacting so positive to the treatments considering the stage of the cancer and the many other chronic health issues. In my opinion, as I have said all along and my endocrinologist tells me every time he says goodbye, "It's in God's hands!" That is something I can live with for as long as God decides my time on this earth is worthy.

When you are living with cancer, or any other health condition that can take your life such as heart problems, blood clots, sarcoidosis or any of the other many diseases which are life threatening, you can develop a different mindset about life. I have learned to turn another popular saying around to make my life more positive – "Never put off tomorrow what you can do today."

I now put off something for tomorrow every day that I could have done today because for me I have to expect tomorrow to come. Now I make sure (unless I'm having one of those "in bed all day" days) I do what I put off or else I'm just procrastinating and that is not the objective. The objective is to always expect the future to come. I plan for trips and other activities down the road because my mental attitude expects the future to come. I know, and understand, in reality tomorrow is not promised to anyone and one day tomorrow will not come for me. However, living with cancer I do not assume tomorrow will come or hope tomorrow will come. No, I **expect** tomorrow to come every single night I lay my head to sleep. I have no doubt or second thoughts that I will see the sun rise once again! It is an attitude critical to your mental success in dealing with any health condition that can take your life, or otherwise.

Before I close I want to stress something I have stressed many times in the past. Always keep your teenagers, children, or grandchildren, aware of the truth of your health condition and let them be involved as well. Of course the level in which you inform and involve them depends on many factors such as the maturity of the individual and putting it in a way they understand as opposed to scaring or worrying them. Here is a perfect example regarding my, at the time, 2 year 8 month-old granddaughter.

On October 29, 2008 I had my PICC Line removed and a port inserted just under my skin in my upper right chest, which was just a more convenient way of having my chemotherapy received. My granddaughter loves to jump on me while I'm sitting down and lay her head on my chest. She also likes for me to pick her up. When I had my port inserted I was under strict weight limitations as to what I could pick up and like with all minor procedures that require cutting you open and stitching you up, it hurt and was sore for a few weeks. So obviously during this time picking up my granddaughter, having her jump on me or laying her head on the right side of my chest was off limits. But how was she to know that or that it wasn't because of something she did wrong?

When she first came over and immediately went to have me pick her up, my wife told her, "No, PaPa can't pick you up now." She looked confused as I leaned down and gave her a hug. When I was sitting down she, as usual, ran up to me and was ready to jump on me when again my wife said, "You can't jump on PaPa right now." My granddaughter looked at me as to ask, "What did I do wrong?"

So I had her sit down beside me and I pulled my shirt down and showed her the incision/stitches. She looked at it and asked, "Hurt?" I replied, "Yes, PaPa went to the doctor today. That's why I can't pick you up or have you sit in my lap right now. But don't worry it will be okay soon and then I can pick you up again!" "Okay" she said in a hope you get better soon tone of voice.

For the next couple of weeks one of the first things she would do when I sat down was to get next to me and pull down my shirt to look at the incision spot, which also bulged where the port is in place. She would ask, "Hurt?" and I would reply, "No, it's getting better." For which she would ask, "You okay?" and I would say, "Yes." She would then give me a kiss, tell me she loved me, and go about her business of having fun.

Gradually she would get in my lap real careful and make sure she stayed on my left side as she would repeat her process of looking and questions/replies. She would even catch herself when she was about to move her head to my right side, as she would get sleepy. She would still lift her arms for me to pick her up but seemed to be satisfied when I bent down and gave her a hug.

Finally on Thanksgiving I was all healed up and picked her up for the first time during the afternoon while we had company in the house. That evening after everyone had left (she spent the night with us that night) she got in my lap once again and brought on another one of those tearjerker moments that makes life so great. She pulled my shirt down and touched the port and asked, "PaPa, you okay now?" I replied, "Yes, PaPa is okay." She looked at me with a big smile and said, "You can pick me up now!" then turned to my wife and said, "PaPa can pick me up now!" I looked at her and said, "Yes, I can pick you up now. PaPa missed picking you up." She again smiled at me and said, "Me too PaPa! I love you!" then gave me a big kiss, before kissing her own hand and putting it on her lips as to her kissing herself as I told her, "I love you too Saniya." She then looked at me with those granddaughter eyes and put her head on my right shoulder for the first time as if to say, "PaPa's back!" I must admit I was grabbing a tissue to wipe a tear from my eye as my heart felt that warm feeling only a grandchild can invoke.

She likes to watch and help me take my medications as well. Before eating she will help me with my insulin by taking off the top of the insulin pen (which is basically like a writing pen and poses no danger to her) and hold it while I put the needle on and inject myself, as she watches every movement from a few steps away. Then after I take the needle off and secure it she will replace the top on the pen, help me put it in the refrigerator, then give a big smile as she says, "I did it!"

She will also sit across the table from me while I take my many pills and watch my every motion as I take each pill. I'm one of those people who regardless of how big or small the pill is I can only take one at a time. There was one night when she was staying with us that I had got my six before bedtime pills and was going to the kitchen to take them, as she was watching TV. Next thing you know I heard her little footsteps come running to the kitchen yelling, "Wait PaPa, wait PaPa!" When she got to the kitchen she climbed up on the seat, looked at me and said, "Okay PaPa, go ahead." I couldn't do nothing but laugh as she watched me take every pill.

The message to these stories are she, even at her young age, understands that her PaPa feels bad sometimes just like she does and it is not her fault when this happens. Children and teenagers will blame themselves when things they don't understand, like health issues that are hidden from them, occur to the adults they love and the adults cannot do with them what they normally do. Don't put your children in a bubble because one day that bubble will burst.

In closing I want to say that, in my opinion, the most important factors in dealing with chronic health conditions such as sarcoidosis or cancer, along with my 3-Step Philosophy described earlier in this book, is to remain positive about your situation, no matter how difficult that might be, and keep a strong faith in your beliefs. I cannot stress enough the importance of a positive attitude and how it will affect every aspect of your life! Learn to appreciate even the bad days. I don't know where my life is going from here, none of us do, not even the healthy. You can only live your life to the best of your ability with the faith that God, or in whatever you personally believe, will take care of you. I strongly feel with the love and unconditional support of my wife, who gives me reason to wake up every morning regardless of how I feel, the inspiration of my granddaughter, the treatments I'm receiving, the support from my daughter, mother, family and friends, the many prayers from people I don't even know, and most importantly, my unconditional faith in God – I'll be okay. Death is inevitable so do not fear it but instead embrace life as you know it.

When I wrote my first book I titled it, *Me & Sarcoidosis – A Lifetime Partnership*. The reason was first there was me, and then came sarcoidosis, for which we are partners for life. I guest now my title should read, *Me, Sarcoidosis, & Cancer – A Lifetime Partnership…To Be Continued*. Life is what it is and none of us has control over the plan God has for us. We must take care of our health in order to take care of others. Do all you can to stay healthy!

If I can leave you with just one thought, remember this. If I can deal with sarcoidosis, the multitude of chronic health conditions I live with on a daily basis, and cancer in a positive manner…if my wife can continue to put up with me while maintaining her other responsibilities she now must deal with successfully…if I can continue to maintain positive relationships with my medical family and loved ones …and if I can continue, despite those bad days from time to time, to maintain a positive attitude towards life – you can as well. There is nothing special or extraordinary about my life, about me or my wife. Don't use us as an inspiration – use yourself and those others in your life. I'm only an imperfect human being and a patient just like you! Your inspirations are all around you, not on TV or in books! Sometimes your inspirational hero is not seen nor heard or for that matter could be taken for granted. They might not hit you in the face or be the obvious, but instead you have to sometimes look a little harder. True inspiration comes from the heart and is not intended to draw attention but instead bring whatever is needed to you at this time in your life. It's the little, but yet important, things in life that count. Life itself is the ultimate blessing! Cherish every moment and everyone in your life!!! Stay positive and healthy…it's the only way to live!

...16...

Please support sarcoidosis and cancer awareness, research, and patient support. And please, as a patient, don't forget the caregivers and your loved ones, they are our lifelines. It's up to each one of us to make a difference. Are you up for it?

Acknowledgments
From The Author

To My Mother – Georgia Barr…My Wife – Ma-Shelle Barr…&…My Daughter – Ra-Shelle Thomas:

There are no more words that haven't already been said or written that can express how important the three of you are to my life. What else can I say except, "Thank you for putting up with me and I love all of you deeply for eternity!"

To My Aunt Dean & Uncle Wayne Spradley:

You are two very special people who provide unconditional love and support to our entire family and those you love. I'm blessed to have you both in my life and I love you both dearly! PS: Nobody gives fish fries like the two of you do!

To Marjorie Woodell:

Thank you for taking the time to help with my manuscript and the valued advice. I learned so much from you during this process. You said it was a labor of love, and with all sincerity, the love is returned!

To Everyone Who Has And Does Support Me:

Thank you to everyone, those of you who I know and those of you who I don't, that sent me e-mails, cards, posted messages on message boards, and any other media used to communicate your support during my current battle with cancer. I especially want to thank everyone who took the time to include me in your prayers. I could never truly express how much your support and prayers mean to me, therefore I'll just say, "Thank You!"

To Everyone Who Has And Does Support My Wife:

Thank you to everyone, in both her business and personal life, who supports my wife/caregiver during my current battle with cancer, sarcoidosis and the many chronic health conditions that affect her life on a daily basis. You all have had such a positive impact regarding the many added physical responsibilities and emotional ups and downs she must endure, which in turn, has made my life more positive as well.

Last, But Not Least, To My Granddaughter – Saniya Marie Akins:

You are the inspiration of my life. Words cannot come close to expressing the feelings of love you give me with everything you do. Always remember that even though one day I might not be around, I will always be with you and looking over you forever! I love you as only a PaPa can – unconditionally and with all of my heart/soul!!!

You can contact Gilbert Barr, Jr. @...

WWW.GILBERTBAR-RJR.COM

Thank You For Your Support

Gilbert Barr, Jr.